YOUR CHILD HAS SCOLIOSIS

Now What Do You Do?

Options to stay ahead of the curve

Cover Design by Siniša Poznanović
Typesetting by Eled Cernik

Dr. Andrew Jay Strauss
250 West Route 59, Suite 4
Nanuet, New York, 10954
USA

For more information:

Contact the Author
(845) 624-0010
www.HudsonValleyScoliosis.com

or

CLEAR Scoliosis Institute
(866) 663-7030
www.clear-institute.org/

ISBN 978-0-9975789-2-8

Printed in the United States of America

Second Edition, November, 2016

Disclaimer

Contents

I. SCOLIOSIS – WHAT YOU NEED TO KNOW

II. WHAT CAUSES SCOLIOSIS?

III. SCOLIOSIS TREATMENT

Acknowledgements

My most deep hearted thank you to all my patients and their families over the past 35 years of practice. It was my incredible good fortune to find my profession. When I look back on the immense responsibility that so many thousands of parents have entrusted in me I am truly humbled, and driven to continue to increase my skills and knowledge. I am very fortunate to have many colleague's that I consider to be friends in the world of conservative scoliosis care and I am grateful for their insights and shared passion which has helped me along my journey as a scoliosis clinician. I apologize in advance for not listing them all. A few individuals played a major role in making this book a reality. My first thanks go to Dr Steven Raposo who urged me into this project and patiently and tirelessly worked with me until completion. Throughout he has been generous with his encouragement and expert advice. Along with thanks to my clinical team, Dawn Rooney, Darleen Haupt, Alex D'Onofrio, Cinnette Wilder, Marcus Brownlee and Dr Marie Janvier, I must single out Heather Rooney my personal assistant. Her dedicated assistance and keen editorial vision has been essential to the completion. I know she has always seen this book as a very personal project and I truly appreciate her commitment to scientific rigor. Thank you to Drs Josh and Dennis Woggon for your review and suggestions on the CLEAR Scoliosis Institute information. Thank you to my nephew Tyler Strauss and his significant other Ashton Schwarz for the excellent pictures of Ashton performing yoga postures. Thank you to my illustrator, Abdul Mannan. You were very patient and never refused the numerous revisions I asked of you. My daughters Zaria and Yekira suffered through many days and nights missing their father while he was in his study working on this book, thank you! My son, Gabe who offered support and key moments of insight and advice. My wife, Elle, went through a lot and did a lot – I would have given up long ago without her steady support, wisdom, and endless patience. My ultimate gratitude goes to the Holy Blessed One who has orchestrated all.

Preface: Introduction

Do You Want to Stabilize – and Even Reduce – Your Child's Scoliosis without Ineffective, Uncomfortable and Outdated Braces or Painful, Potentially Disabling Surgery?

Of course you do!

And, so do I. In 35 years of practice, I have helped thousands of scoliosis sufferers improve their conditions and take back control of their lives.

Scoliosis can be a very scary and traumatic condition.

You find out that your child's spine is curving too much. You slowly realize that the problems can grow worse as they get older. The only scoliosis treatment options presented to you have been the traditional ones, and they are not very satisfying. You can either:

1. Watch and wait/do nothing and hope the scoliosis doesn't get worse *(really the opposite of a treatment option)*

2. Have your child wear an ineffective brace for up to 23 hours per day that – at best – will only stabilize the condition. *(Often this makes the scoliosis worse.)*

3. Undergo invasive scoliosis surgery to stabilize and possibly fuse metal rods to your child's spine with risk of dangerous complications and the need for additional follow-up operations.

Few people realize that these options only treat the symptoms of scoliosis, but not the real cause.

You could go from specialist to specialist seeking opinions without ever knowing that there is an alternative treatment for the condition, one shown to be effective in stabilizing and reducing scoliosis curves and minimizing – even eliminating – pain by addressing the *CAUSE* of scoliosis.

Who Am I?

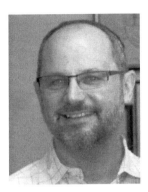

Dr. Andrew Strauss, BS, MS, DC

My journey to become a chiropractic doctor started with my own personal experience with chiropractic's healing power as a young child. In my youth, my health was destroyed by regular and severe chest pain. My family consulted traditional medical specialists, but nothing relieved my excruciating discomfort.

It wasn't until my family ignored traditional medicine and tried chiropractic care that I experienced a phenomenal cure for this debilitating pain. At that point, I made the decision to devote my life to providing the health-restoring healing art of chiropractic.

I graduated with a Bachelor of Science in Biology with honors from the University of New Hampshire in 1978. I went on to study chiropractic at Palmer College of Chiropractic in Davenport, Iowa, the world's oldest and largest chiropractic college. I graduated with honors in 1982.

I have a master's degree in acupuncture from the Royal Melbourne Institute of Technology, a Doctorate in Traditional Medicines from Medicina Alternativa, and a graduate diploma in Chinese herbalism. Other postgraduate training has included advanced studies in spinal mechanics, exercise physiology and clinical nutrition, as well as courses in various physical therapies and diagnostics such as computerized traction, whole-body vibration, foot orthotics, manipulation under anesthesia, laser acupuncture, scoliosis bracing design, electromyography and radiology.

All of this paved the way for my work in the field of scoliosis treatment, a vocation that has now spanned 35 years. After studying spinal biomechanics with Dr. Dennis Woggon in the early 1980s, I continued working closely with him and the CLEAR Scoliosis Institute to gain its highest level of certification. I am the vice president of CLEAR, a nonprofit scoliosis institution and am on its technique advisory committee. I am a member of the Palmer College of Chiropractic Alumni Association, past president Upper Cervical Society, and member American Academy of Spine Physicians.

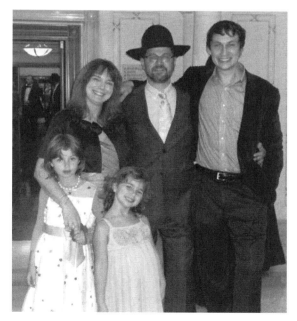

On a personal note, I am married to Elle,
and we have two daughters and a son.

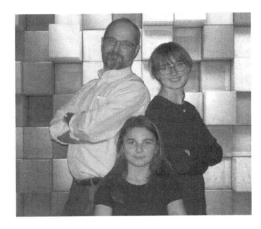

In my work, I've seen the physical and emotional trauma caused by scoliosis and have made it my mission to treat and reduce scoliosis cases. In most instances, I have been able to accomplish this without the use of braces or surgery. My practice, the Hudson Valley Scoliosis Correction Center in New York, offers conservative and natural healing focused on the treatment of scoliosis. This book is a natural outgrowth of my mission to serve scoliosis patients by educating them and their families about the treatment alternatives available to them.

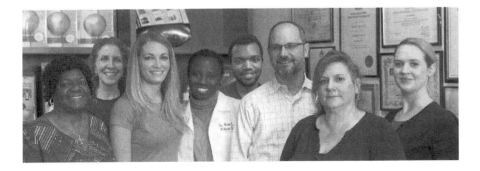

My staff and I utilize a wide variety of chiropractic techniques, an American science more than 100 years old; modern applications of Chinese medicine, which dates back 3000 years; and clinical nutrition and wellness practices, which have stood the test of time. Combined with a wide knowledge and application of new evidence based exercise-based treatment strategies for scoliosis care from all over the world AND the very latest evolution of scoliosis bracing, these things are providing dramatic help for scoliosis sufferers.

The newer techniques work well because they target the root cause of scoliosis rather than just treat the symptoms. By seeking to maximize the natural strengths of the body and its capacity to heal itself, I am able to help patients help themselves.

I've found that orthodox medicine most commonly recommends dealing with scoliosis symptoms in three ways – none of which actually treat the underlying cause.

Bad Option No. 1 – "Observe" The Scoliosis and Do Nothing

It is common practice for doctors to recommend "observing" mild scoliosis curves, also called a "watch and wait" approach. What this really boils down to is once the scoliosis is discovered, it is re-x-rayed until it progresses past a 20-degree curve. Then, the "observing" doctor states that the patient is a candidate for either bracing or possibly even surgery. (*I devote a whole chapter in this book to surgery, explaining why it should be seen only as a last-resort treatment choice.*)

Bluntly, "watch and wait" is not a scoliosis treatment; it is just doing nothing and hoping the scoliosis won't get worse. It will.

> *Patients come in saying, "It was just a mild scoliosis curve until all of a sudden it just took off and progressed over 40 degrees. Now my doctor is recommending spinal fusion surgery!"*

Bad Option No. 2 – Use Outdated Scoliosis Braces That Are Ineffective

For more than 500 years, the back brace has been around as a treatment for scoliosis. (You will get to read a detailed account of its invention and adaptations in Chapter 22.) Yet until very recently, there has been no definitive evidence of its effectiveness. The goal of scoliosis bracing was always stabilization, not correction. All too often, a scoliosis brace even fails at that!

Scoliosis braces such as the Boston Brace, the Milwaukee Brace, the Providence Brace, the Charleston Brace and countless others around the world are ill-fitting and are designed to lock the scoliosis into its distortion. This is similar to what a cast does to a broken arm; it locks the bone into place. This does not work with scoliosis and is seen by many as just "a waiting room for surgery." You will learn why bracing can only be effective when it is accompanied by a scoliosis specific exercise program that has been custom designed for the patient.

Most scoliosis braces are not designed to correct curves. Older design scoliosis braces will attempt to hold the spine in place so the curve doesn't get any worse. Modern designs can be corrective when utilized skillfully.

Bad Option No. 3 – Have Highly Invasive Scoliosis Surgery with Potentially Dangerous Complications

The most common scoliosis surgery is highly invasive and requires doctors to make a large incision down the back. The ribs are spread, and one or more steel alloy rods are inserted along with hooks, pins and pieces of bone to secure the remaining bones and fuse the spine into place to prevent further curvature. This procedure is followed by a painful recovery period that leaves patients with large scars.

A 2002 German study on the long-term quality of life for idiopathic scoliosis patients who had received Harrington instrumentation, reported "40 percent of operated treated patients with idiopathic scoliosis were legally defined as severely handicapped persons."[1] That's scary.

---

1 Götze, C. et al. «[Long-term Results of Quality of Life in Patients with Idiopathic Scoliosis after Harrington Instrumentation and their Relevance for Expert Evidence].» *Zeitschrift fur Orthopadie und ihre Grenzgebiete* 140.5 (2001): 492-498. 18 Apr. 2016

However, this book's purpose is not meant to make you anxious. It's meant to calm the minds of patients and their parents. Scoliosis is the subject of much research, and knowledge is power!

By educating yourself about scoliosis, you'll be able to make informed choices about the best treatment option for you. You also will be able to determine which type of care you should accept first and which treatment options should be your last resort in almost any scenario.

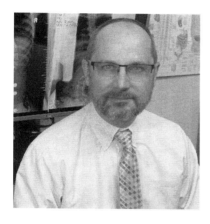

Yours in health,

Dr. Andrew Strauss, BS, DC, MS

P.S. Remember that all severe scoliosis curves have one thing in common; they started out as mild curves and progressively got worse. Do something about your child's scoliosis N-O-W and reclaim control over your family's life.

> "Nature is the source of all true knowledge. She has her own logic, her own laws, she has no effect without cause nor invention without necessity."
>
> — Leonardo da Vinci

I. SCOLIOSIS – WHAT YOU NEED TO KNOW

Chapter 1. The World of Scoliosis: Definitions and Diagnosis

Hippocrates, the ancient Greek physician, first wrote of spine deformity in 460 B.C. Approximately five centuries later, the Greek physician Galen introduced specific terms for normal and abnormal spinal curves. He coined medical terms such as **"scoliosis," "kyphosis"** and **"lordosis."** The word "scoliosis" comes from a Greek word meaning "crooked." So essentially, scoliosis means "crooked back" or "crooked spine." The healthy spine has normal curves when looking from the side, but it should appear straight when looking from behind.

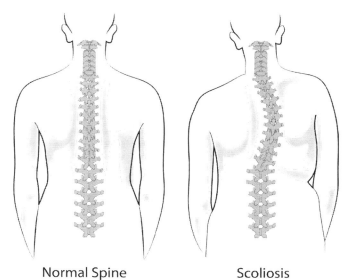

Normal Spine   Scoliosis

Scoliosis a term used to describe a spine that has twisted abnormally to the side. Kyphosis is a curve seen from the side in which the spine is bent forward. There is a normal kyphosis in the mid back, or thoracic spine region. Lordosis is a curve seen from the side in which the spine is bent backward. There is normal lordosis in the cervical spine and the lumbar spine.

People with scoliosis develop one or more additional curves to the sides, and the bones of the spine twist on each other, forming C-shaped or S-shaped curvatures. It may or may not be noticeable to others.

Experts classify scoliosis as:

- **Nonstructural scoliosis** (also called "functional scoliosis"): the spine is structurally normal, and the curve is temporary. A typical cause for this type of scoliosis is muscle spasm causing temporary postural changes.

- **Structural scoliosis:** the spine has a structural problem. The cause could be a variety of neurologically based or muscle-based diseases; injuries to the spine, legs or pelvis; infection of the bones; birth defects; a short leg; or most commonly "idiopathic" causes, which is medical jargon meaning "no known cause."

"Why Do People Get Scoliosis?"

Scoliosis **"etiology"** (study of a disease's cause) holds mostly unanswered questions. In most people, there is no known reason for development. This is known as **"idiopathic scoliosis."** This is the most common type of scoliosis seen in children 7 years of age through their early teens – when children are growing fast.

Small curve idiopathic scoliosis is equally common in girls and boys. Larger curves are much more common in girls than boys. It can be seen at any age, but it is typically first noticed in those older than 10 years of age. Scoliosis can present in people of all ages. About four out of every 100 children have some form of scoliosis.

Scoliosis can run in families, and modern theories suggest a genetic link. A child who has a parent, brother, or sister with idiopathic scoliosis should be screened regularly for scoliosis. Physicians use medical and family history, physical exam and genetic tests when checking a person for scoliosis. An x-ray of the spine will confirm if a person has scoliosis. The scoliosis x-ray lets the doctor measure the angle of the curve in degrees and see its location, shape and pattern.

"Is Scoliosis Painful?"

In the large majority of cases, scoliotic curves in children will not cause pain. If the curve is greater than 30 degrees, the curve may get worse in adulthood with pain developing between 30 and 50 years of age and beyond. If there is pain present, treatment should always be designed to alleviate pain first, then stop curve progression, reduce curve size, and stabilize the curve corrections.

All large scoliosis curves have one thing in common; they started as small curves! It is much easier to treat a smaller-sized scoliosis and effectively reduce the curve, preventing curve progression and the associated pain and disability. If you or a family member have a smaller curve, get it corrected before it has a chance to develop into a larger curve. Why watch and wait until it becomes larger?

Chapter 2. How to Tell if Your Child Has Scoliosis

Often, scoliosis is first noticed by a friend or family member. Since changes in the spine happen gradually and always begin as a smaller curve, it may go unnoticed by the individual. As the curve becomes more severe, individuals will begin to notice that their clothes do not fit the same or that pant legs are shorter on one side than the other.

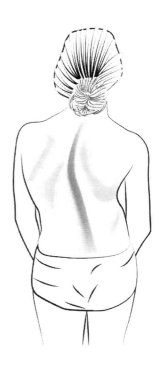

The most common sign of scoliosis is an abnormal curve of the torso. While a healthy spine has a natural curvature when viewed from the side, it appears as a straight line when viewed from the back. However, an individual with a significant scoliosis will appear to have a side-to-side curve in their spine when viewed from behind.

What to Look Out For

Scoliosis may cause the head to appear off center or one hip or shoulder to be higher on one side of the body. Your child may have a more obvious curve on one side of the rib cage from the twisting of the vertebrae and ribs.

If scoliosis sufferers bend forward to touch their toes, thoracic curves will make one shoulder blade stick out prominently. Curves in the lumbar region of the back will show very little evidence of their existence when bending forward. If the scoliosis is very severe, it can make it difficult for the heart and lungs to work properly. This can cause shortness of breath and chest pain.

There are certain types of scoliosis that can cause back pain. When back pain is present with scoliosis, it may be because the curve in the spine is causing stress and pressure on the spinal discs, nerves, muscles, ligaments or facet joints. Whether your child has any back pain associated with scoliosis or not, it is very important that they see a doctor to find out what is causing any pain they may experience.

Signs of Scoliosis

In children and teens, scoliosis often does not have any noticeable symptoms. The curvature of the spine often does not cause pain, and if the curve is mild, it can go unnoticed. Even without an x-ray of the spine, there are several common physical signs that may indicate scoliosis. It is not uncommon for it to be discovered during a routine school examination for scoliosis in states that mandate scoliosis screening.

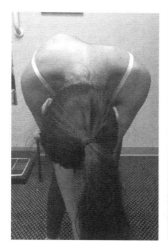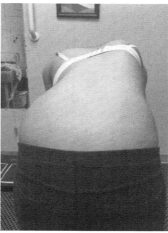

Adam's Forward Bend Test

One of the most common tests for detecting scoliosis is called the **Adam's Forward Bend Test** in which the individual bends from the waist as if touching her toes.

Although there are often few noticeable signs of scoliosis, screeners look for one or more of the following indicators:

Scoliosis Symptoms and Signs in Children

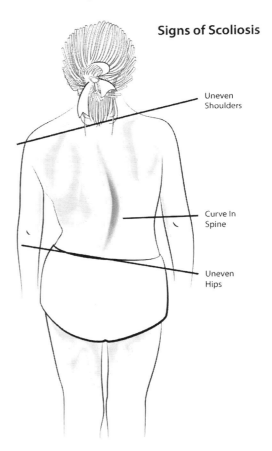

Signs of Scoliosis

Uneven Shoulders

Curve In Spine

Uneven Hips

- Shoulders may not be the same height (one higher than the other)

- Head is not centered directly above the pelvis

- Rib cage is not symmetrical (ribs may be at different heights)

- One shoulder blade is higher and more prominent (it sticks out)

- One hip is more prominent (higher) than the other

- The individual may lean to one side

- One leg may appear shorter than the other

- The waist appears uneven

- Clothes do not fit or hang properly

- On the Adam's Forward Bend Test, one shoulder blade will protrude

A tool called a "scoliometer" is used to quantify the amount of curve.

If you suspect your child has scoliosis or have noticed any of the telltale signs, it is important to have an exam conducted by a scoliosis professional for proper diagnosis and possible treatment options.

> "In the long run, we shape our lives, and we shape ourselves. The process never ends until we die. And the choices we make are ultimately our own responsibility."
>
> - **Eleanor Roosevelt**

Chapter 3. The Many Forms of Scoliosis

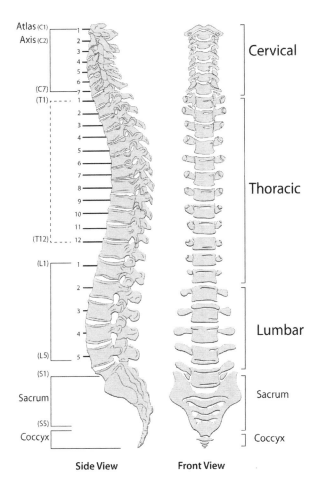

Side View   Front View

Scoliosis is not a disease, rather the word is a term used to describe any abnormal, sideways or **lateral curvature** of the spine. Viewed from the back, a typical spine looks straight. If the spine curves, it can show up as a curve to either side. It can be a single curve shaped like the letter C — or *"C-shaped scoliosis"* — or the spine can have two curves, resembling the letter S — or *"S-shaped scoliosis."* In rare cases, the spine contorts into triple and quadruple curves.

The spine has 24 vertebrae that are divided into three sections: **cervical** (the seven vertebrae of the neck), **thoracic** (the 12 vertebrae of the middle back), and **lumbar** (the five vertebrae of the lower back).

Scoliosis can occur in the neck (**cervical spine scoliosis**), in the middle back (**thoracic spine scoliosis**) and in the lower back (**lumbar spine scoliosis**) in various combinations.

For example, a lumbar curve typically involves a curve to the left in the lower back that affects an average of five vertebrae. **Thoracolumbar scoliosis** is curvature that includes vertebrae in both the lower thoracic and upper lumbar portions of the spine. Scoliosis that involves both the thoracic and lumbar spinal regions are called **"double major curves."**

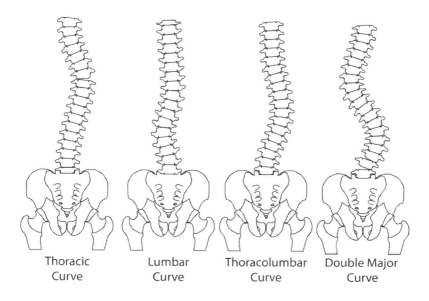

| Thoracic Curve | Lumbar Curve | Thoracolumbar Curve | Double Major Curve |

Common Scoliosis Terms Explained

Dextroscoliosis is a spinal curve to the right ("dextro" means right). Usually occurring in the thoracic spine, this is the most common type of curve. It can occur on its own (forming a C-curve) or with another curve bending the opposite way in the lower spine (forming an S-curve). The reason a right-hand or "dextro" thoracic scoliosis is most common is that the body instinctively avoids the heart which is located to the left of the midline of the torso.

Levoscoliosis is a spinal curve to the left ("levo" means left). Common in the lumbar spine, the rare occurrence of levoscoliosis in the thoracic spine indicates a higher probability that the scoliosis may be secondary to a some kind of disease or illness such as a spinal cord tumor or **chiari syndrome**.[2] Chiari malformation means part of the cerebellum is entering the opening at the base of the skull instead of staying in the skull. In the case of a levoscoliosis in the thoracic spine, an MRI study often is recommended.

Kyphosis is a forward-bending curve of the spine, when seen from the side. There is a normal kyphosis in the middle (thoracic) spine, but if the spine is bent excessively forward, it is classified as a **kyphotic spine**. This may sound confusing, but when the thoracic spine is referred to as kyphotic on a report, that is always due to excessive kyphosis as there would be no references to this with normal findings.

Kyphoscoliosis is an abnormal curvature of the spine consisting of *both* kyphosis and scoliosis.

Lordosis is a curve that — when seen from the side — features a spine bent posteriorly or backward in the cervical neck region and the lower back lumbar area.

---

2 "Chiari Malformation Fact Sheet." 2006. 23 Mar. 2016 <http://www.ninds.nih.gov/disorders/chiari/detail_chiari.htm>

"How Can the Most Common Type of Scoliosis Have No Known Cause?"

The type of structural scoliosis that has no known cause occurs in approximately 4 percent of children. Research shows adolescent idiopathic scoliosis (AIS) affects 1-3 percent of children in the at-risk population: 10-16 years age.[3] When we add in those children younger than 10, we arrive at the figure of 4 percent. If we include adult numbers in our calculations, the incidence percentage is much higher.

As mentioned previously, the term "idiopathic" means a condition or disease with no known cause. Idiopathic scoliosis is by far the most common cause of scoliosis. Vast amounts of research have been done over many years to determine what causes it, but at the time of this writing there is no definitive answer. Many theories have been put forward. Yes, most scientists will agree that there is a genetic connection, but what triggers the expression of these weakened genes is still a puzzle. Don't be surprised; there are many conditions that are not fully understood.

Medical science is making steady progress on figuring scoliosis out. Risk factors that are linked to causing the genetic expression of scoliosis present themselves in many forms. The technical word for this is "epigenetics." Some of the possible factors include trauma to the spine, exposure to certain bacteria types, hormonal imbalances, bad posture from heavy backpacks, or even nutritional deficiencies. At the time of the writing of this book, there have been 47 different things implicated in either the development or the progression of scoliosis. We can assume that there are many more that will become apparent as more research continues to be done.

---

3 Weinstein, S.L. "PubMed — NCBI." 2008. 26 Apr. 2016
<http://www.ncbi.nlm.nih.gov/pubmed/18456103>

Idiopathic scoliosis rarely causes pain. Once scoliosis is detected, it should be closely monitored by a scoliosis professional who will initiate a proactive plan to ensure the curve does not progress and — if possible — will be reduced and stabilized. Active custom-designed exercise therapy prescribed by a scoliosis expert is currently recognized as the best starting point for mild curves.

To More Fully Understand Scoliosis, Let's Look at the Types of Idiopathic Scoliosis

Idiopathic scoliosis has been somewhat artificially divided into three sub-groups according to age: *infantile* (0-3 years), *juvenile* (4-10 years), and *adolescent* (11- maturity). Once maturity is reached, it is then classified as *adolescent scoliosis in an adult (ASA)*.

Please keep in mind that if the scoliosis started in a 3-year-old, but was not identified until the child was 11, it could still be referred to mistakenly as "adolescent scoliosis." This is a big problem when attempting to make sense of the development of scoliosis. But, let's still take a look at this classification system anyway.

Infantile Idiopathic Scoliosis – Yes, Babies Can Have Scoliosis!

Infantile scoliosis is defined as scoliosis that is first diagnosed in a child between birth and 3 years of age. Ninety percent of early onset scoliosis will resolve without treatment.[4]

Those that do not resolve can be difficult to manage. Frequent checkups are needed, and if progression is seen, aggressive non-surgical treatment must be started. The child will not be able to benefit from an exercise-based

---

4 "Infantile Scoliosis — Medscape Reference." 23 Mar. 2016 <http://emedicine. medscape.com/article/1259899-overview>

program at this age. The best forms of care start with either serial plaster casting or the use of hard plastic hyper-corrective bracing methods. There is currently a variety of invasive surgical methods based on the insertion of expandable rods used for treating infantile scoliosis.

Juvenile Idiopathic Scoliosis: Age 4–10

Juvenile onset scoliosis is defined as spinal curves diagnosed between ages 4–10. It is less common than adolescent scoliosis but still makes up about 10–15 percent of all scoliosis cases.[5] I have found children of this age to benefit from exercise-based care programs. Success rates are high with proper coaching from a dedicated doctor and his staff when combined with the help of a well-trained parent, guardian or even a school teacher. A team approach is best.

Adolescent Idiopathic Scoliosis: Tweens and Teens

Adolescent idiopathic scoliosis (AIS) occurs in children ages 11–maturity and comprises approximately 80 percent of all cases of idiopathic scoliosis. This age range is when rapid growth typically occurs, which is why a curve at this stage should be monitored closely as the child's skeleton develops. This is when there is the highest risk of progression. Sometimes in this age group the new over-corrective bracing is necessary. The advanced designs are effective, and patients are often very motivated to perform the home-exercise routines to avoid surgery. Adolescents are old enough to understand the choices they are making and typically want surgery ONLY as a last resort!

Adolescent Scoliosis in an Adult

Once skeletal maturity is reached, a patient with adolescent idiopathic scoliosis is now said to have adolescent scoliosis in an adult (ASA). A patient with ASA will benefit greatly from treatment for progression. Pain unfortu-

---

5 Wick, JM. "Infantile and Juvenile Scoliosis: The Crooked Path to …" 2009. 25 Apr. 2016 <http://www.aornjournal.org/article/S0001-2092(09)00551-1/abstract>

nately has become a common reason to seek treatment. Normal degenerative changes of the spine may be accelerated by the scoliosis curvature and the patient may be at higher risk for skeletal pain or extremity pain due to nerve compression.

Yes, Adults Get Scoliosis, Too!

Not to be confused with adolescent scoliosis in an adult (ASA), **adult scoliosis** – or a**dult onset scoliosis** – is a degenerative scoliosis, which is side-to-side curvature of the spine caused by degeneration of the spinal joints. Degenerative scoliosis shows up in middle age and older adults, most frequently in people aged 35–65. Typically a C-shaped curve forms in the lumbar spine. It can occur due to wear and tear causing osteoarthritis in the spine, or "spondylosis." Weakening of the normal ligaments and other soft tissues of the spine combined with abnormal bone spurs can lead to an abnormal curvature of the spine.

The spine can also be affected by osteoporosis, vertebral compression fractures, and disc degeneration. These changes and their associated pain cause individuals to lean to one side to reduce pressure causing spinal deformity. Degenerative scoliosis is the most common form of scoliosis in adults and is often seen in those who had a milder form of scoliosis as a child. Please see my second book entitled, Adult Scoliosis, expected to be published in early 2017.

Types of Scoliosis for Which We Know the Cause

Structural scoliosis presents as a fixed curve and is treated case by case. It can be caused by a variety of neurological and/or muscular disorders or birth defects such as hemivertebra, in which one side of a vertebra fails to form normally before birth. It also can result from leg length discrepancies, metabolic diseases, connective tissue disorders, rheumatic disease, or injury to the spine, legs or pelvis.

The vertebrae can fail to form completely or fail to separate from each other during fetal development. This type of scoliosis develops in people with other disorders, (i.e. birth defects, muscular dystrophy, cerebral palsy, or Marfan's disease). People with these conditions often develop a long C-curve. Their muscles are just not able to hold their spines straight.

Nonstructural (functional) scoliosis: Nonstructural scoliosis is a curve in the spine without rotation. It is reversible because it is caused by a treatable condition such as pain, muscle spasm or a difference in leg length. In this type of scoliosis the spinal curvature is a healthy adaptation to a temporary problem.[6]

Compensatory scoliosis: This spinal curve disappears when the patient sits. It may be caused by either a short leg, misshaped pelvic bones, or a pelvic tilt due to hip contracture. This type of curve will straighten significantly with side-bending to produce spinal balance. Compensatory scoliosis can be caused by a misalignment of the spine ("vertebral subluxation" or "pinched nerve"). Often, this type of scoliosis can be treated with great success by a general practice chiropractor.

The location of the **structural curve** determines the classification of the scoliosis. For example, a 12-year-old with a structural curve of unknown cause in the thoracic spine is called "thoracic adolescent idiopathic scoliosis." The exact definition of the curve has implications for determining scoliosis progression and scoliosis treatment.

This is an explanation of a few basic terms used to classify scoliosis. If it appears complicated, it is. Don't make the mistake of assuming you have enough understanding to self-diagnose. There are even more complicated classifications for scoliosis such as the Rigo, King and Lenke classification systems.[7]

It's always best to consult your physician who has expertise in scoliosis with any questions you may have about your scoliosis diagnosis.

---

6 "Scoliosis Causes & Types (Structural & Nonstructural)." 2007. 24 Mar. 2016 <http://www.webmd.com/back-pain/tc/scoliosis-cause>

7 "Lenke Classification System for Scoliosis | Lawrence Lenke ..." 2012. 24 Mar. 2016 <http://spinal-deformity-surgeon.com/a-leader-in-spinal-deformity/lenke-classification-system-for-scoliosis/>

Chapter 4. Roundback (Kyphosis)

There are normal and abnormal spine curves. Although the spine should be straight when viewed from behind or from the front, it should exhibit normal mild curvature when it is viewed from the side.

In a healthy back, the cervical (neck) and lumbar (low back) segments of the spine are curved slightly. **"Kyphosis"** comes from the Greek word for "hump." Excessive curvature of the thoracic (middle) spine is known as "kyphosis" or the common terms **"roundback"** or **"hunchback."**

The individual bones or vertebrae that make up a healthy spine look like squares stacked in a column. Kyphosis occurs

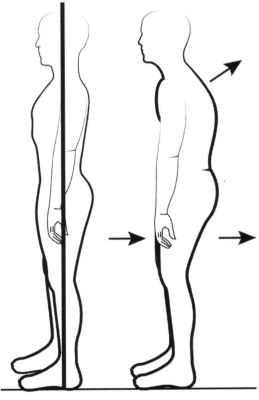

Good Posture   Thoracic Kyphosis / Hunchback

when the vertebrae in the upper back become more wedge shaped, curving the spine and causing the spinal column to lose some — or all — of its lordotic profile. This causes a bowing of the back, seen as a slouching posture.

While most cases of kyphosis are mild and only require routine monitoring, serious cases can be debilitating. High degrees of kyphosis can cause a distressing cosmetic deformity as well as severe pain and discomfort, breathing and digestion difficulties, cardiovascular irregularities, neurological compromise, and even significantly shortened life spans in the more severe cases.

Types of Kyphosis

Postural kyphosis is the most common type and can be found in children and adults. In childhood and adolescence, it is commonly attributed to slouching and is reversible by correcting muscular imbalances. In older patients, it is referred to as "**hyperkyphosis**" or "**dowager's hump.**" It indicates a Cobb angle greater than 40 degrees and is most common in older women. If the curve angle exceeds 70—75 degrees, many surgeons will recommend a complex surgery to reduce the kyphosis. Hyperkyphosis can develop due to aging alone, but about one-third of the most severe hyperkyphosis cases occur after osteoporosis weakens spinal bones to the point that they crack and compress.

Scheuermann's kyphosis is a significantly worse deformity. It can cause varying degrees of pain and can also affect other areas of the spine — most commonly the mid-thoracic region.

More commonly referred to as "**Scheuermann's disease,**" it is found mostly in teenagers. Boys are affected more often than girls. A patient with Scheuermann's kyphosis cannot consciously correct posture because the apex of the curve is very rigid. The patient may feel pain at this apex, which can be aggravated by physical activity and long periods of standing or sitting. Whereas the vertebrae and disks appear normal in postural kyphosis, these structures in Scheuermann's kyphosis are irregular, often herniated, and wedge-shaped over at least three adjacent levels.

Fatigue is a very common symptom, most likely because of the intense muscle work required to stand or sit properly. The condition appears to be hereditary. Most of the patients who undergo surgery to correct their kyphosis have Scheuermann's disease.

Congenital kyphosis manifests in rare cases in which an infant's spinal column does not develop correctly in the womb. Vertebrae may be malformed or fused together and can cause progressive kyphosis as the child develops. Surgical treatment may be necessary at a very early stage, and consistent follow-up will be an important part of maintaining a normal curve. However, the decision to carry out the procedure can be very difficult due to potential risks to the child. A congenital kyphosis also can appear suddenly in teenage years — more commonly in children with cerebral palsy and other neurological disorders.

Nutritional kyphosis can result from deficiencies in the diet, especially during childhood. A vitamin D or calcium deficiency, for example, can cause rickets, a softening of the bones that results in curving of the spine and limbs under the child's body weight.[8]

Gibbus deformity is a form of structural kyphosis, where one or more adjacent vertebrae become wedged. Gibbus deformity can result from advanced skeletal tuberculosis and is caused by collapsed vertebral bodies. This can lead to spinal cord compression causing paraplegia, an impairment in motor or sensory function of the lower extremities.

Post-traumatic kyphosis occurs from untreated or ineffectively treated vertebral fractures.

Kyphosis Diagnosis

For kyphosis diagnosis, a physical examination is required. A health care provider will check height and may ask the patient to bend forward from the waist while he or she views the spine from the side. The rounding of

8 Sahay, M. "Rickets–Vitamin D Deficiency and Dependency — NCBI." 2012. 26 Apr. 2016 <http://www.ncbi.nlm.nih.gov/pmc/articles/PMC3313732/>

the upper back may become more obvious in this position. Reflexes and muscle strength will be checked, and depending on symptoms, x-rays may be ordered. These tests will help determine the degree of curvature, if there are any deformities of the vertebrae, and to identify the type of kyphosis if it is present. If there is numbness or muscle weakness, the doctor may recommend tests to determine how well nerve impulses are traveling between spinal cord and extremities. If the kyphosis is severe, the doctor may check for breathing interference using **"spirometry,"** a lung function test.

Kyphosis Treatment

Kyphosis treatment depends upon age, cause and effects. Kyphosis also may cause back pain and stiffness in some people. Mild cases of kyphosis may produce no noticeable signs or symptoms. Stretching exercises can improve spinal flexibility in cases of **postural kyphosis**. Exercises that strengthen the abdominal muscles may help improve posture, too. In many older people, kyphosis is a sign of osteoporosis, the loss of bone density and strength. It has a variety of causes.

The discomfort and strain of structural kyphosis can be helped by performing specific mobilizing exercises, sensorimotor re-integration maneuvers, and a kyphosis brace which may be prescribed to be worn all day or possibly only at night. The program of care can in most cases improve spine mobility and reduce postural distortions, as well as prevent progression. In selected pediatric and adult patients, there can be a modest reduction in the overall size of the kyphosis.

If the kyphosis curve is severe, particularly if the spinal bones are pinching the spinal cord or nerve roots, surgery may be prescribed. Spinal fusion surgery connects two or more of the affected vertebrae permanently. Surgeons insert bits of bone between the vertebrae and then fasten the vertebrae together with metal wires, plates and screws. The complication rate for spinal surgery is relatively high, and problems may include bleeding, infection, pain, nerve damage, arthritis, and disk degeneration. Followup surgeries may be needed.

Chapter 5. Swayback (Lordosis)

Remember that a normal spine, when viewed from behind, appears straight. From the side, the spine normally curves at the neck, the torso, and the lower-back area. This positions the head over the pelvis naturally. These curves also work as shock absorbers that distribute the stress that occurs during movement.

Normal spinal contours are essential for the correct biomechanics of the spine. Nature designed the spine as a marvelous machine combining the strength of a column with the flexibility of a spring.

Lordosis is the inward curvature of a portion of the lumbar (low back) and cervical (neck) spine. In a spine affected by **hyperlordosis,** or **excessive lordosis,** the vertebrae of the low back are curved, giving a swayback appearance.

A major factor of this spinal distortion is **anterior pelvic tilt**, when the pelvis tips forward when resting on top of the femurs (thigh bones). When lying on your back on a hard surface, a large degree of lordosis will appear as a space between the lower back and the surface.

Excessive lordosis may increase at puberty, although it is sometimes not evident until the early or mid-20s. Excessive lordosis, or **hyper**lordosis, is commonly referred to as "**hollow back**," "**sway back**" or "**saddle back**," a term that originates from the similar condition that arises in some horses.

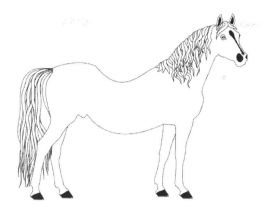

A reduction in the normal lower-back curve is called "**hypo**lordosis."

This loss of normal lordosis will cause a stretching of the disc posteriorly, compressing it anteriorly and potentially causing a narrowing of the opening for the nerves, possibly pinching them.

Symptoms of Swayback

Hyper (too much) or **Hypo** (too little) lordosis can lead to moderate to severe lower back pain and can cause pain that affects the ability to move. If the curve is flexible (reverses itself when the person bends forward), there is little need for concern. If the curve does not change when the person bends forward, the lordosis is fixed or locked, and treatment is needed.

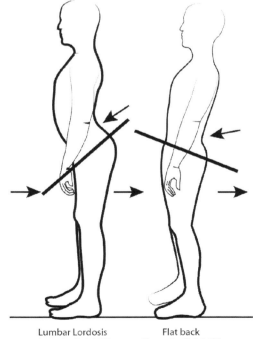

Lumbar Lordosis
/ Anterior Pelvic Tilt
/ Swayback

Flat back
/ Posterior Pelvic Tilt

Causes of Lordosis

Hyperlordosis affects people of all ages. It is common in dancers and gymnasts, and certain conditions can contribute to lordosis, including, kyphosis, pregnancy, osteoporosis and excessive belly fat. A heavy belly may pull the pelvis to the front, tilting the spine too much. Imbalances in muscle strength and muscle length are also a cause. Tight lower back muscles, weak hamstrings and overly tight hip flexors may aggravate the condition. Rickets, a vitamin D deficiency in children, also can cause lumbar **hyper**lordosis.

Hypolordosis is commonly found in adolescent idiopathic scoliosis (AIS) patients.

Lordosis Diagnosis

To diagnose lordosis, the patient's medical history and a physical exam are necessary, especially if excessive or diminished curve becomes noticeable or seems to be getting worse. The patient will be asked to bend forward and to the side to see whether the curve is flexible or fixed, how much range of motion the patient has, and if the spine is aligned properly. The doctor may feel the spine to check for abnormalities.

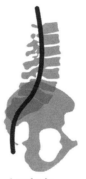 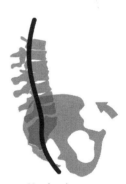

Lordotic
Lumbar Spine

Kyphotic
Lumbar Spine

A neurological assessment may be necessary if the person is having pain, tingling, numbness, muscle spasms or weakness, sensations in his or her arms or legs, or changes in bowel or bladder control. X-rays may be taken of the whole back or just the lower back.

Treatment for Lordosis

Lordosis treatment involves building strength and flexibility to increase range of motion. **Lumbar lordosis treatment** consists of strengthening muscles on the back of the thighs and stretching the group of muscles on the front of the thighs. The muscles on the front and on the back of the thighs can rotate the pelvis forward or backward while in a standing position because they can discharge the force on the ground through the legs and feet.

Back hyperextensions on an exercise ball will strengthen posterior muscles and help lordosis. Sensorimotor re-integration techniques are used to target the problem and retrain the brain to hold the corrected posture. This is done by placing weights on the body while standing on an unstable surface like a foam mat or a balance disc.

Clinicians have found that it is not uncommon for hypolordosis to accompany scoliosis. This may be due to instability in the spine caused by lack of the normal curve. Part of scoliosis care must be to protect and augment the normal spinal contours.

Scoliosis surgery and the older clam shell-type scoliosis braces are problematic because they can worsen the loss of normal curves in both the neck and back, which then weakens the spine. The newly developed, customized, three-dimensional scoliosis braces support and encourage normal curves of the spine, whereas "off the shelf" older brace designs may diminish or fail to restore normal curves.

Hypolordosis can be corrected non-surgically through rehabilitation exercises. If done correctly, symptoms can be reduced in three to six months. If excess belly fat is contributing to the **hyper**lordosis, then weight loss may be required to decrease the curve. Only the most severe cases of lordosis require surgery, which may involve spinal instrumentation, artificial disc replacement, and kyphoplasty – the surgical filling of an injured or collapsed vertebra.

As with AIS, early detection is key to treating lordosis.

> *"We must let go of the life we have planned, so as to accept the one that is waiting for us."*
>
> **- Joseph Campbell**

Chapter 6. Infantile Scoliosis

Early onset scoliosis, or infantile idiopathic scoliosis, is defined as scoliosis that is first diagnosed in a child between birth and 3 years of age. Parents usually first notice that their child persistently lies in a "banana shape" or sits leaning to one side. A prominence of the ribs on one side of the back or chest may be seen or felt. Infantile idiopathic scoliosis occurs in two basic types: resolving and progressive.[9] About 20 percent of infantile idiopathic scoliosis cases do not resolve and can be difficult to manage.[10]

Often magnetic resonance imaging (MRI) is used to determine if there are any abnormalities of the spinal cord or spinal column. Sedation or general anesthesia is needed to relax the child enough to obtain quality images.

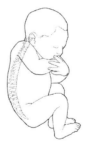 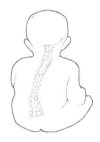

Many infantile curves are left-sided curves in the thoracic (middle) spine, whereas they occur more commonly on the right side in adolescent idiopathic scoliosis. Many infants are otherwise healthy and just have a small curvature of the spine. In some infants, however, there is an increased association with hip dysplasia, mental retardation and congenital heart disease.

9 "Casting and Traction Treatment Methods for Scoliosis (PDF ...)" 2015. 21 Apr. 2016 <https://www.researchgate.net/publication/5900787_Casting_and_Traction_Treatment_Methods_for_Scoliosis>

10 Sengupta, DK. "Scoliosis – The Current Concepts." 2010. 26 Apr. 2016. <http://www.ncbi.nlm.nih.gov/pmc/articles/PMC2822419/>

Congenital scoliosis (caused by malformed and/or connected vertebrae) also is diagnosed during this period. However, these curves are not included in the infantile idiopathic scoliosis category. Congenital scoliosis forms during the first six weeks of embryonic formation.[11]

Scoliosis fusion surgery isn't used in infantile scoliosis because the spine and lungs aren't mature; they need to fully develop. A fusion would prevent further growth of the instrumented segment of the spine.

Also, depending on the type of instrumentation used, the anterior spine may continue to grow leading to "crankshaft phenomenon." This occurs when the front part of the spine is fused, and the spine twists as it grows. In this situation, the infantile scoliosis continues to progress despite the posterior fusion. For this reason, other surgical treatments have been developed for the management of early-onset scoliosis. These techniques take into account the spine's growth, as well as the growth of the rib cage and lungs. If implants are prescribed, multiple surgical expansions or lengthenings may be needed (usually twice per year) to keep up with spine growth.

It is typically advised that parents wait three to six months to determine whether or not the scoliosis will progress. This is one place "watch and wait" is sometimes appropriate. However, there is a measuring technique used with infantile scoliosis to help determine if the curve is progressive or self-resolving. The rib vertebral angle degree (RVAD) is measured and analyzed to indicate what type of curve is present. Because maximum correction and curve resolution depend on the time in which treatment is administered, the sooner treatment is started the better and the greater the chance of success.[12]

---

11 "Patients and Families — Scoliosis Research Society." 2015. 25 Mar. 2016 <https://www.srs.org/persian/patient_and_family/scoliosis/index.htm>

12 "Rib Vertebral Angle in Scoliosis | Bone and Spine." 2013. 25 Mar. 2016 <http://boneandspine.com/rib-vertebral-angle-in-scoliosis/>

Serial Casting

The most commonly used early treatment involves serial corrective plaster scoliosis casts. Serial casting is now the medical treatment of choice to be used in children with infantile scoliosis.[13]

Early treatment with serial corrective plaster EDF (elongation, derotation, flexion) jackets/casts is a preventive treatment that is provided as soon as an infant's scoliosis is considered progressive. The infant's curve will keep pace with the child's growth rate, which is about 24 centimeters in the first two years. Depending on how quickly the child is growing, casts are changed approximately every two 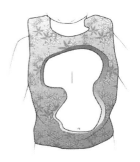 months for children younger than 2, around every three months for those aged 3 years, and every four months for children 4 years and older.

Plaster of Paris is typically used for the scoliosis cast. It doesn't dry as fast as fiberglass, allowing time to address rotation and apply the most effective correction. A fiberglass layer is applied on the outside of the cast to protect the plaster. A large cutout in the front of the cast allows the child breathing room and provides rib flaps to support the rib cage and prevent permanent rib flaring. There is another cutout in the back that is trimmed on the concave side of the scoliosis curve. This cutout allows the flattened ribs on the concave side of the curve to grow out and the prominent ribs on the convex side to grow flat. The child is recast every two to six months as growth occurs. There is now a rigid plastic brace that can be used for infantile scoliosis. It is a fully padded, over-corrective, hard plastic brace. Yes, it is more expensive to replace the hard plastic brace than the plaster cast as the child grows, but the plastic brace can be removed, allowing for baths and playtime.

13 Canavese, F. "Serial Elongation-derotation-flexion Casting for Children with ..." 2015. 1 May 2016 <http://www.ncbi.nlm.nih.gov/pmc/articles/PMC4686440/>

> *"Youth is the spirit of adventure and awakening. It is a time of physical emerging when the body attains the vigor and good health that may ignore the caution of temperance. Youth is a period of timelessness when the horizons of age seem too distant to be noticed."*
>
> **- Ezra Taft Benson**

Chapter 7. Adolescent Idiopathic Scoliosis

Adolescent idiopathic scoliosis (AIS) (sometimes referred to as **"teenage scoliosis"**) is defined as a lateral or side-to-side curvature of the spine greater than 10 degrees and accompanied by vertebral rotation. It is present in 2–4 percent of children between 10-16 years of age.[14] It may start even before puberty and dramatically increase during a growth spurt.

Though the cause is unknown (idiopathic), most researchers affirm that genetics are associated with the condition. Not all adolescents diagnosed with scoliosis have curves that progress. The likelihood of curve progression can be estimated in some cases using genetic testing. Genetic testing has been called into question lately and the findings must be considered in the context of the whole case.

Scoliosis curves smaller than 10 degrees are present in both girls and boys equally, but girls outnumber boys 10 to one[15] when curves are greater than

---

14 Reamy, BV. "Adolescent Idiopathic Scoliosis: Review and Current Concepts." 2001. 26 Apr. 2016 <http://www.ncbi.nlm.nih.gov/pubmed/11456428>

15 Reamy, BV. "Adolescent Idiopathic Scoliosis: Review and Current Concepts." 2001. 26 Apr. 2016 <http://www.ncbi.nlm.nih.gov/pubmed/11456428>

30 degrees.[16] Scoliosis tends to progress more often in girls than in boys. This is because girls have their growth spurt when they are younger and less posturally mature. Boys catch up to the girls in height when they are older. The boys' postural centers in the brain have had more time to develop, placing them at a lower risk for scoliosis progression.[17]

Teenage scoliosis is most often discovered during a routine physical exam. Pain is not typical in adolescent scoliosis and if present may indicate some other condition contributing to the scoliosis.[18]

Here are two interesting facts that must be considered when a teen with scoliosis has back pain.

1. Research has shown that 70-80 percent of adolescents will get intermittant back pain.[19]

2. Research has shown that some where between 6-20 percent of teens with scoliosis have back pain.[20]

So...the child or teen with scoliosis AND back pain may have two unrelated issues with her spine!

Let's review what signs to look for when scoliosis is suspected:

*   Shoulders may not be the same height

*   Head is not centered above the pelvis

16 Reamy, BV. "Adolescent Idiopathic Scoliosis: Review and Current Concepts." 2001. 26 Apr. 2016 <http://www.ncbi.nlm.nih.gov/pubmed/11456428>

17 Negrini, S. "Why do we treat adolescent idiopathic scoliosis ... — NCBI." 2006. 22 Apr. 2016 <http://www.ncbi.nlm.nih.gov/pubmed/16759352>

18 "Evaluation of Back Pain in Children and Adolescents ..." 2009. 11 Apr. 2016 <http://www.aafp.org/afp/2007/1201/p1669.html>

19 Jones, G. "PMC Free PDF — NCBI — National Institutes of Health." 2005. 26 Apr. 2016 <http://www.ncbi.nlm.nih.gov/pmc/articles/PMC1720304/pdf/v090p00312.pdf>

20 Ramírez, Norman et al. "Back Pain During Orthotic Treatment of Idiopathic Scoliosis." *Journal of Pediatric Orthopaedics* 19.2 (1999): 198-201. Print.

- Ribs may be at different heights

- A shoulder blade may stick out

- The individual may lean to one side

- One leg may appear shorter

- The waist appears uneven

- Clothes do not fit/hang properly

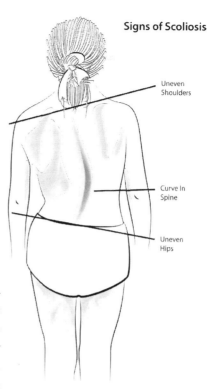

Signs of Scoliosis

Uneven Shoulders

Curve In Spine

Uneven Hips

"How is Scoliosis Diagnosed?"

If the scoliosis is in the upper back, a physical examination will reveal a more prominent shoulder blade when the child or teen bends forward. You may recall that this is called an "Adam's forward bend test." Often the spine curves to the right in the upper back and to the left in the lower back, causing the right shoulder to be higher than the left. If the scoliosis is in the lower back, one hip may be more prominent than the other. X-rays taken while the child or teen is standing will confirm the extent and type of scoliosis.

Traditionally, adolescent idiopathic scoliosis was only treated with scoliosis bracing. Surgery was the next option if the curve was deemed at a high risk of progression. Smaller less severe curves were only monitored and treated when they became large and more severe.

That Was Then. This Is Now!

Now, there is a more proactive approach than the previous wait-and-see method. It is important to treat scoliosis curves **BEFORE** they progress rather than **AFTER**. Not only are there more treatment options that address scoliosis early on, but there are also non-invasive treatments that do not employ the use of scoliosis braces.

Modern home care programs use custom-designed scoliosis exercises consisting of spinal resistance training in
conjunction with the principles of specific brain-retraining maneuvers to restore the spine's alignment. Adolescent
scoliosis patients are further treated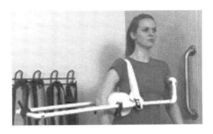
with a customized sensorimotor re-integration program that includes treat-
ment on various machines combined with scoliosis exercises. Early intervention is essential to reduce the curve and avoid the difficulties inherent in
large-curve treatment.

While scoliosis treatment programs (including exercise-based, bracing or surgery) may not eliminate scoliosis completely, they will reduce and stabi-lize the curve. It is fine for the child to enter adulthood with a mild scoliosis and continue to use a custom-designed home exercise program as they con-tinue to age. This gives them the power to control the condition themselves.

First, use a custom-designed, scoliosis specific exercise-based home program. Then consider the hyper-corrective bracing along with the exercise program. Only as a last resort should the patient submit to a surgical correction.

This just makes sense!

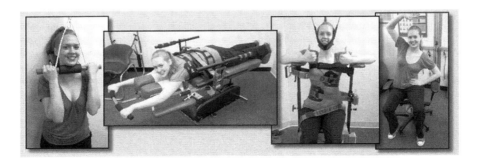

> *"From a small seed a mighty trunk may grow."*
>
> **- Aeschylus**

Chapter 8. Let's Talk About Children With A 'Mild Scoliosis'

Mild scoliosis is a 10- to 20-degree curve, when assessed by Cobb Angle. Mild Scoliosis has a 22 percent chance of progressing, which is significant risk. Once the scoliosis passes the 20-degree mark, risk of progression more than triples to 68 percent!

Symptoms of Mild Scoliosis

- Scoliosis curve is less than 20 degrees

- May have tilted head, uneven shoulders or hips

- Head may appear more forward than shoulders when viewed from the side (forward head posture)

- Clothing may hang unevenly

- May have uneven leg lengths.

- May not be observable from posture, even by pediatricians or school screeners

- May or may not be accompanied by pain

- Mild scoliosis is found equally in girls and boys.

- (Large curves are found ten times more often in girls vs. boys.)

Mild Scoliosis Treatment

- Easier to treat when the curve is small

- Overwhelmingly the research shows that mild curves respond well to exercise-based correction without the need of bracing in most cases. To achieve this impressive result, it is vital to remove the "drivers" of the scoliosis before the 30 degree mark occurs. The appropriate custom designed program of spinal cord stretching, neurological re-education, along with isometric and isotonic exercises will maintain the upper hand against the forces underlying curve progression.

- Genetic testing using a saliva sample can determine how likely the curve is to reach surgical threshold (please see Chapter 16 to understand the nature of genetic testing for scoliosis)

"All **LARGE** Scoliosis Curves Have One Thing in Common.
They Started as SMALL Curves."

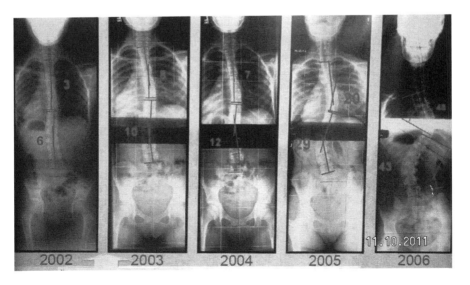

Why Early Scoliosis Intervention is Crucial

It can be nearly impossible to tell just by looking at a person whether or not they have scoliosis. This is often the case for mild scoliosis patients. Patients often contact my office will a similar tale of being unaware of their child's scoliosis for years. While scoliosis appears to be a side-to-side curve in the spine, it is actually a twisting of the spine around its axis causing the rib cage to rotate as well. This twisting of the spine can gradually cause a severe torque that makes the existing spinal curve twist and bend even more. The effect becomes visible when the torso is pushed to one side causing a "rib hump." These postural changes can even occur before the Cobb angle measurement indicates a problem. When treatment is initiated while the curve is still small there is a far greater chance of reducing the curve to 10 degrees or less.

Chapter 9. What Adulthood Looks Like for a Child with Scoliosis

Once skeletal maturity is reached, a patient with adolescent idiopathic scoliosis is now labeled as having **adolescent scoliosis in an adult (ASA)**.[21] There would typically be a slow increase (about 0.5-1 degree per year) in the curvature[22] that began during teen years in an otherwise healthy individual which is progressive during adult life.[23]

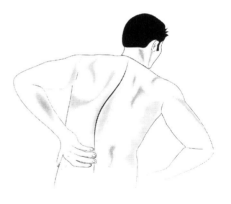

These curves can occur in the thoracic (upper) and lumbar (lower) spine and have the same basic appearance as those seen with adolescent scoliosis. Physical symptoms can include: shoulder asymmetry, a rib hump, or a prominence of the lower back on the side of the curvature.

21 "Adults with Idiopathic Scoliosis Improve Disability ... — Springer." 2016. 11 Apr. 2016 <http://link.springer.com/content/pdf/10.1007%2Fs00586-016-4528-y.pdf>

22 Negrini, A. "Scoliosis-Specific Exercises Can Reduce the Progression of ..." 2015. 26 Apr. 2016 <http://www.ncbi.nlm.nih.gov/pmc/articles/PMC4537533/>

23 "PubMed Result — NCBI." 2014. 26 Apr. 2016 <http://www.ncbi.nlm.nih.gov/pubmed?link_type=MED_NBRS&access_num=3182881&cmd=Link&dbFrom=-PubMed&from_uid=3182881>

Though an adult with adolescent scoliosis will still benefit from adult scoliosis exercises to stop progression, now pain is a much more universal reason for treatment. Commonly, patients were diagnosed with idiopathic scoliosis earlier in life, but were not prescribed treatment because their curves were not deemed severe enough to warrant the standard medical approach of bracing or surgery. These patients later find that by adulthood their curves have either progressed so that they now require treatment or now are causing pain. Other patients may have been braced with the older brace designs during adolescence only to have their "corrected" curves revert or continue to progress as adults.

Adult scoliosis patients differ from adolescent patients because the curves tend to cause back pain – often the main complaint. The curves also tend to be rigid, more severe and progressive, making treatment more challenging. Advanced stages of disc degeneration are also associated with adult scoliosis and may be the primary reason for back pain in many patients. Pinched nerves from herniated discs and arthritic changes may also be a challenge. In late middle age and after, it is common for patients to develop osteopenia (low bone density) or osteoporosis – factors which affect treatment. Because normal degenerative changes of the spine may be accelerated by curvature, the older patient may be at higher risk for skeletal pain or extremity pain from nerve compression. So, even though a child's curve may appear insignificant or symptomless, preemptive treatment helps the patient avoid more difficulty as they age.

It is important to have a specialist in adult scoliosis monitor the curve because these curves can worsen due to the disc degeneration. This also may cause patients to lean progressively forward. This forward shift in posture is the greatest predictor of pain and disability in adults with scoliosis. Also, arthritis in the spine facets can lead to bone spurs, pain and stiffness of the back. In more severe cases, it can lead to shooting pain and numbness down the legs from pinched nerves.

> *"Pregnancy and motherhood are the most beautiful and significantly life-altering events that I have ever experienced."*
>
> **- Elisabeth Hasselbeck**

Chapter 10. Pregnancy and Scoliosis

"Will Scoliosis Interfere with My Child's Fertility or Future Efforts to Carry a Baby to Term?"

Since idiopathic scoliosis is common in girls, there are concerns about the effects it may have on pregnancy or becoming pregnant. Over the past 40 years, several studies have been conducted with hundreds of women who showed **NO** difference in pregnancy, labor, delivery and fetal complications – whether they had scoliosis or not.

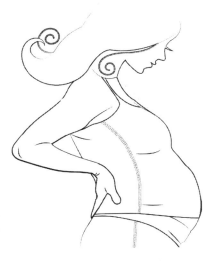

There is **NO** evidence that scoliosis reduces fertility or leads to an increased number of miscarriages, stillbirths or congenital malformations.

Scoliosis does not have an adverse effect on becoming pregnant or the ability to deliver full-term children – even in extremely large-curve cases.

"What About Pregnancy Potentially Causing a More Rapid Progression of the Curve?"

Another major pregnancy concern is increased risk of progression of the scoliosis. Some studies have shown that patients lost 2, 6 and 18 degrees of correction during their first pregnancies, but curves stayed the same or improved with later pregnancies. So, while there can be a time of curve progression during pregnancy, generally scoliosis does not increase during pregnancy. As long as the curve is not in a progressive phase, the weight gained during pregnancy does not increase the curvature.

Aside from a mild degree of restricted lung capacity, individuals with idiopathic scoliosis rarely experience breathing problems during pregnancy, unless there is a pre-existing lung condition or impairment. Breathlessness on exertion is a common complaint in the early months of pregnancy for all women.

Shortness of breath is partly caused by the rise in progesterone, which stimulates breathing by increasing respiratory rate and the depth of each breath. Blood volume also increases. These normal physiological changes are well tolerated and only likely to be problematic if the vital capacity is low or heart function is compromised. Scoliosis that occurs in the middle spine may affect breathing. Bladder and bowel problems may be an issue for women with scoliosis who already have urinary or bowel dysfunction.

Back Pain and Scoliosis During Pregnancy

Physical health and pre-existing back problems can affect the amount of back pain experienced when pregnant. It's been stated that as many as 40 percent of women who have had their scoliosis surgically corrected experience increased low back pain during pregnancy.[24] However, many women with *no* abnormal curvature still have mild to moderate back pain during pregnancy, so it can be difficult to distinguish whether the pain is from the scoliosis or pregnancy. Maintaining a good fitness program and addressing existing back problems prior to pregnancy may help mothers avoid or reduce back discomfort.

---

24 Orvomaa, E. "Pregnancy and Delivery in Patients Operated by the ... — NCBI." 1997. 26 Apr. 2016 <http://www.ncbi.nlm.nih.gov/pubmed/9391799>

Pregnancy and Severe Scoliosis

Women with severe scoliosis (over an 80-degree Cobb angle) should consult their doctor before becoming pregnant as some cases may require monitoring of the scoliosis and fetus. Also, because the uterus pushes the diaphragm higher and decreases capacity, some breathing problems may be experienced during the later stages of pregnancy. Health care providers may choose to manage these respiratory problems by prescribing non-invasive positive pressure ventilation through a CPAP. Back pain can also be significant for pregnant women with severe scoliosis, compared to non-scoliotic patients.

Pregnancy and Congenital Scoliosis

Individuals with congenital scoliosis or early-onset scoliosis and those with weak muscles and heart problems should seek medical advice before becoming pregnant. Congenital scoliosis is often associated with neuromuscular conditions such as muscular dystrophy or poliomyelitis. These are genetic and some can be detected prenatally.

Breathing will also be affected if the muscles that expand the rib cage are weak. Lung size may also be more severely restricted because of certain birth defects. Evidence suggests that as long as the vital capacity exceeds around 1.25 liters, the outcome will probably be good. Below this level, problems with a reduction in oxygen worsen on exertion and during sleep and may be accompanied by a rise in carbon dioxide levels. Low oxygen levels are harmful for the growing baby and also can lead to heart strain in the mother. CPAP ventilation machines have been used to guard the health of mothers and facilitate the birth of healthy, full-term babies.[25]

To ensure a healthy pregnancy, scoliosis patients need to follow the guidelines for proper nutrition, rest, exercise, prenatal medical and chiropractic care as outlined by their obstetricians. Patients also should see their scoliosis specialists regularly to monitor curve status.

---

25 Allred, CC. "Successful Use of Noninvasive Ventilation in Pregnancy." 2014. 25 Apr. 2016 <http://err.ersjournals.com/content/23/131/142.full.pdf>

Chapter 11. Relieving a Child's Scoliosis Pain

"I Thought Scoliosis in Children Wasn't Painful!"

The absence of any pain associated with scoliosis is an identifying hallmark of a diagnosis of adolescent idiopathic scoliosis. The presence of pain is considered an important clinical indicator that the scoliosis may be a symptom of some underlying issue such as tumors, infection, disc herniation, spinal cysts, scars, abdominal muscle spasms, or traumatic injury. In adolescent scoliosis, severe pain is concerning and may indicate the mentioned abnormalities to the spine and musculature. Pain is not a typical symptom of adolescent scoliosis; however, it is commonly associated with adult scoliosis.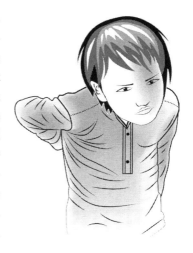

"Can Scoliosis Cause Back Pain?"

Idiopathic scoliosis is a spinal deformity, but it does not typically cause severe back pain. As we discussed earlier, a very large percentage of adolescents with scoliosis experience no back pain, but up to 80 percent of teens will experience intermittent back pain. Individuals with scoliosis can develop back pain, just as most of the adolescent and adult population can develop back pain. However, there is only a small amount of research to suggest that people with idiopathic scoliosis are any more likely to develop back pain than the rest of the population.

Interestingly, studies have shown lower back pain in children and adolescents, just as in adults, is a common condition. Some have shown a lifetime prevalence as high as 70–80 percent by 20 years of age. One study reported 32 percent of patients with presumed idiopathic scoliosis had pain; of these study participants, nine percent were found to have an underlying pathology.[26] [27] [28]

Adult Scoliosis Back Pain

Unlike children, pain is often a common problem reported by adults with either adult degenerative scoliosis (also known as "de-novo scoliosis" or "adolescent scoliosis in an adult" [ASA]). Activity-related musculoskeletal pain is much more common in adults with moderate to severe scoliosis. The adult spine undergoes degenerative changes, which reduce water content in the discs and produce inflammation in the joints. Nerve impingement or "pinched nerves" may occur as a result of a disc herniation. Another source of pain is arthritis of the facet joints.

"What Can I Do About My Child's Scoliosis Pain?"

Scoliosis Exercise Programs

It has been known that the deep core muscles of the spine are primarily controlled automatically by a constantly monitored group of sensors in the

---

26 Calvo-Muñoz, Inmaculada, Antonia Gómez-Conesa, and Julio Sánchez-Meca. "Prevalence of Low Back Pain in Children and Adolescents: a Meta-Analysis." *BMC Pediatrics* 13.1 (2013): 1. 18 Apr. 2016

27 Ramirez, Norman, Johnston, Charles E., and Browne, RIchard H. "The Prevalence of Back Pain in Children Who Have Idiopathic Scoliosis*." *J Bone Joint Surg Am* 79.3 (1997): 364-8. 18 Apr. 2016

28 Jones, GT, and GJ Macfarlane. "Epidemiology of Low Back Pain in Children and Adolescents." *Archives of Disease in Childhood* 90.3 (2005): 312-316. 18 Apr. 2016

brainstem, but the effect of discoordinated function between local and global spinal muscles and back pain is just now becoming understood.[29]

Similarly one of the drivers of idiopathic scoliosis is suspected to be primarily a discoordination between the deep core muscles of the spine and is correlated with increased incidence of back pain as well.

Since most of the traditional therapeutic exercise programs for back pain focus on strength, endurance, fitness and functional capacity only, the connection between idiopathic scoliosis and therapeutic exercise for back pain seemed remote. However, a new understanding of neuromuscular discoordination syndromes is starting to provide insight into the relationship between back pain and scoliosis pain.

A 2000 study highlights why "one size fits all" type therapeutic exercise for back pain associated with any structural problem and especially for patients with scoliosis is inappropriate.

"There is considerable variability in the nature and degree of the motor control problems presenting in patients with low back pain. In the future, links may be found between certain variables in the patterns of motor control exhibited by patients with low back pain and the tendency for severity or persistence of the condition.

In the short term, this variability between patients highlights the need for an individual problem-solving approach to the neuromuscular dysfunction in patients with low back pain in the clinical situation."[30]

"Why Does My Child Have More Pain in His Shoulder Than in His Back?"

---

29 Dietz, V. "Proprioception and Locomotor Disorders — UFJF." 2002. 25 Apr. 2016 <http://www.ufjf.br/especializacaofisioto/files/2013/06/Proprioception-and-loco-motor-disorders.pdf>

30 Jull, GA. "Motor Control Problems in Patients with Spinal Pain: a New ..." 2000. 26 Apr. 2016 <http://www.ncbi.nlm.nih.gov/pubmed/10714539>

Scoliosis and Shoulder Pain

When shoulder pain develops, it will most often develop first on the shoulder that is not affected by curvature.

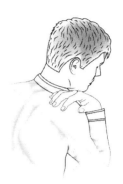

Therefore, if your spine curves to the left, you can expect the right shoulder to show signs of scoliosis shoulder pain first. This is due to the pulling of tendons and muscles as the body tries to overcompensate and pull the spine back into a normal position.

In addition to the initial signs of shoulder pain, as scoliosis progresses without treatment, there is a risk that the other shoulder may begin to experience pain as it bears the weight of the body as the spine curves in that direction. As a result, the shoulder pain will begin to affect the other side, too. This leads to increased disability.

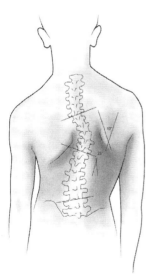

The pain in the shoulders is expected and will continue without treatment.

An exercise-based scoliosis care program can effectively treat many of these types of shoulder pain by balancing the muscles, improving mobility, and most importantly guiding the spine back into a more central posture.

Scoliosis shoulder pain should be considered with all types of scoliosis as a potential health risk. Treatment is necessary to effectively prevent and decrease pain when the shoulders begin to feel the pull of the spinal curvature.

Scoliosis and Hip Pain

While less common than shoulder pain, some children will experience pain in the hips associated with their scoliosis.

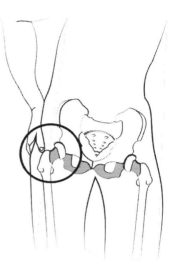

One of the identifying signs of scoliosis is having one hip that appears higher than the other. This can lead to pain when walking or standing for long periods of time. This is postural pain and is caused by the effects of gravity on the unbalanced posture.

Pain is often at the apex of the curve (where the spine curves out the most). Pain develops as a result of ligaments being stretched from spine deformity.

Also, if the pelvis is tilted from scoliosis, then one hip starts to take extra loading, eventually causing severe pain from the overuse/misuse of the tendons and musculature. The pain may subside with rest, but then returns.

Ligament laxity, or looseness, also can cause pain and discomfort. **Sacroiliac joint dysfunction** generally refers to pain in the sacroiliac joint region that is caused by too much or too little motion of the joint. This results in inflammation of the SI joint and can be debilitating. A scoliosis can trigger sacroiliac dysfunction because the weight of the body is shifted to one side, stressing the pelvic joints.

Sacroiliac Joint Pain

The pelvic girdle is made up of the iliac bones and the sacrum (tailbone). The sacrum connects on the right and left sides of the ilia (pelvic bones) to form the right and left sacroiliac joints.

Two major ligaments hold the joints together – the iliolumbar and sacroiliac ligaments. The **iliolumbar ligament** stretches from the top of the right and left iliac crest to its adjacent fourth and fifth lumbar vertebrae. The **sacroiliac ligament** stretches from the sacrum to its adjacent right and left iliac bones.

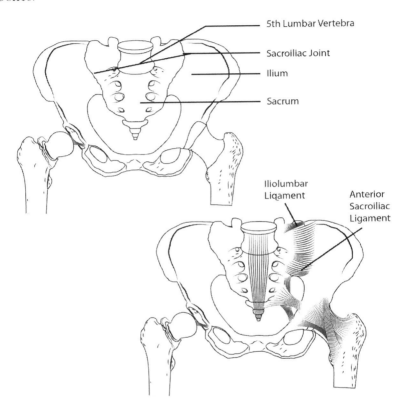

5th Lumbar Vertebra

Sacroiliac Joint

Ilium

Sacrum

Iliolumbar Ligament

Anterior Sacroiliac Ligament

The Many Causes of Sacroiliac Joint Pain

Strain and sprain of the iliolumbar ligament and sacroiliac ligament of the sacroiliac joint are common causes of low back, sacral and other pelvic pain. Sprain to these ligaments is usually due to strain or traumatic injury (e.g. car accident, sports injury, fall). The abnormal postural strain of scoliosis creates long term stresses on the sacroiliac joints and often is the cause of low back pain in the scoliosis patient.

Sacroiliac joint ligament sprain injuries are typically bilateral, meaning they affect both sides, though pain may be more pronounced on one side of the lower back. Lower back pain related to sacroiliac joint ligament sprain is commonly accompanied by misalignment of the sacroiliac joints (usually bilaterally), other pelvic bones, joints and/or the lumbar vertebrae.

Sacroiliac Pain Symptoms

- Low back/groin/buttock pain

- Sciatica (pain down the back of the legs)

- Hip pain

- Increased urinary frequency

- Restricted mobility

- Difficulty walking or twisting

- Difficulty sitting or standing for extended periods

- Temporary numbness, prickling or tingling in the legs/feet

Low back pain from sacroiliac joint dysfunction can be isolated directly over the most problematic sacroiliac joint or both joints. Pain can range from dull aching to sharp and stabbing and increase with physical activity.

Symptoms can worsen after prolonged positions (i.e., sitting, standing, lying down). Bending forward, climbing stairs, walking up a hill and getting up from a seated position also can cause pain. Pain in the leg, groin and hip is referring or reflective pain; the pain is felt in these areas instead of the site of the injury. Often, the ligament pain of SIJ sprain injury spreads or projects in a shooting, radiating pain pattern that often can be confused with "sciatica" of degenerative disc nerve root compression in the older patient. Severe and disabling sacroiliac joint dysfunction can cause insomnia.

Many muscles are connected with the ligaments of the sacroiliac joint including the piriformis. Piriformis syndrome is a condition often related to sacroiliac joint dysfunction. In many cases, there is an associated lumbar vertebral pattern with low-back pain and paralumbar muscular spasm. These muscles can spasm due to a dysfunctional sacroiliac joint.

Pain caused by this joint can refer in many different ways depending on the patient, because the nerves are interconnected. Therefore, patients with sacroiliac joint dysfunction also can develop tightness and dysfunction in the hamstrings, quadriceps, iliotibial tract and hip flexors, including the psoas muscle. Severe and long-standing sacroiliac joint dysfunction can cause muscle deconditioning and atrophy throughout the body due to limitation of activities and exercise that cause low-back pain.

Leg Length Discrepancy

A functionally short leg accompanied by a slight limp and leg abduction (extending the leg out to one side) weakness can be a sign of compensatory scoliosis or an accelerating force causing the scoliosis to become progressive. If your legs are two different lengths, a heel or full sole lift could correct the pelvic tilt and therefore ease some of the extra loading and alleviate some pain.

A 2006 study observed pelvic asymmetry associated with either C-type or S-type scoliosis and found apparent leg-length difference in 87 percent of the patients studied.[31]

Treatment

Sacroiliac joint sprain treatment usually involves treatment of a simultaneous lumbar ligament sprain. A sacroiliac belt may help reduce pain by stabilizing the sacroiliac joint to help maintain reduction of the misalignment and keep the joint in place between treatments.

---

31 Timgren, J. "Reversible Pelvic Asymmetry: an Overlooked ... — NCBI." 2006. 26 Apr. 2016 <http://www.ncbi.nlm.nih.gov/pubmed/16949945>

The presence of a functionally short leg may require treatment with an orthotic device. If the short leg differential is less than 7-10 millimeters (mm),
a heel lift rarely would be used, but a sole lift is needed when the discrepancy is over 10mm. In more extreme cases, the whole shoe may need to be
built up by an orthotist.

"Can Scoliosis be the Cause of My Child's Headaches?"

Up to 50 percent of headaches can be attributed to neck problems. Chronic headaches with neck pain usually involve a
nerve pressure (subluxation) condition
within the neck.[32]

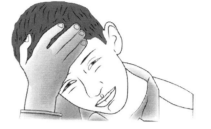

Scoliosis can be associated with a muscle
imbalance in the neck and shoulders,
triggering headache.

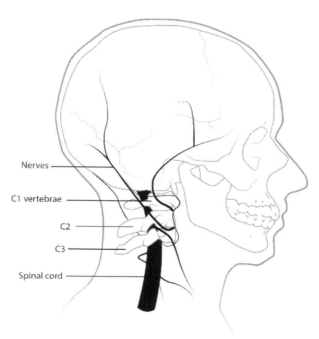

32 Page, P. "Cervicogenic Headaches: An Evidence-led Approach ... — NCBI." 2011.
26 Apr. 2016 <http://www.ncbi.nlm.nih.gov/pubmed/22034615>

Chronic Cervicogenic Headaches

There are seven vertebrae that make up the spine in the neck. These cervical vertebrae surround the spinal cord and canal. Between these vertebrae are discs, and the nerves of the neck pass nearby.

The top three cervical vertebrae are the most likely to refer pain to the back of the head and create a secondary type of headache, called a "cervicogenic headache." Cervicogenic headaches are primarily occipital (at the base of the skull) head pain that originates and is referred from some joint, ligament, muscle, intervertebral disc and/or nerve in the upper neck. There is usually associated pain in the upper neck as well, which is frequently described as "dull," although the pain can become stabbing with head movement.

Causes of Cervicogenic Headaches

Trauma to the Neck

Muscles, ligaments, tendons, joints, discs and nerves of the upper neck can all be injured and cause neck pain, as well as headache. Whiplash from things such as falls, car accidents or athletic injuries cause misalignments in the neck called "subluxations." Poor posture due to scoliosis can function as a low-level, but relentless, micro-trauma to the neck. Any repetitive movements under this stress can cause subluxations, leading to neck pain and headaches.

Muscle Tension in the Neck

There are many muscles in the shoulders, neck and base of the head that can develop tension and inflammation and cause chronic neck and head pains. When neck and scalp muscles become tense and contract from stress, depression, a head injury, and/or anxiety, tension headaches can occur.

Scoliosis causes postural strain and often causes this type of neck muscle tension, which can lead to nerve pressure and tension headaches.

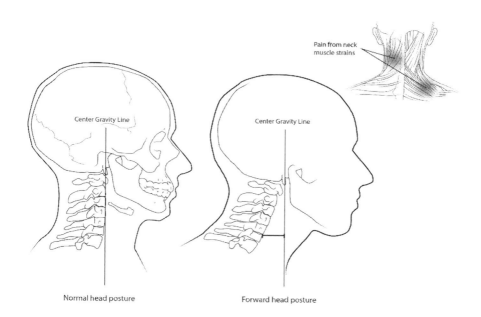

Pain from neck muscle strains

Center Gravity Line

Center Gravity Line

Normal head posture   Forward head posture

Tension headaches are the most common type of headache, and although a band-like constrictive pain around the head is most common, upper neck pain is not unusual. Computer work, stomach sleeping and reading in bed also can trigger tension headaches.

Chapter 12. Scoliosis Assessment

"What is the Doctor Looking for When He Examines My Child?"

We've established that watch-and-wait is a waste of critical time, but how *should* scoliosis be assessed and checked?

The evaluation of a patient should always begin with a comprehensive history and record review, scoliosis examination, and the appropriate x-rays. Assessment might include:

Computerized postural assessment — A digital photograph is analyzed by computer software to precisely measure all postural distortions. This is used as a before-and-after evaluation tool.

Range of motion study — The doctor will ask your child to move his or her spine gently through its complete range of motion to locate areas of restricted or excessive motion.

X-ray evaluation — X-rays of the neck and scoliosis areas will be taken. Special views will be taken if short leg syndrome or other abnormalities of the spine and pelvis are suspected. X-rays are crucial to secure an accurate analysis of the structure of the scoliosis.

Respiratory function assessment — This evaluation utilizes a computerized instrument that the patient blows into. Because certain scoliosis types can impact lung capacity, this test is vital for a full evaluation.

Muscle strength and balance — The key muscles supporting the pelvis and the spine are evaluated for weakness and any side-to-side or front-to-back imbalance.

Coordination and proprioception — These areas are evaluated to determine the appropriate intensity for a custom-designed exercise program. The patient will be asked to balance on one foot, to march in place, and do other maneuvers to evaluate ability to perform home exercises. The program of scoliosis exercises must be individually designed to respect a child's limitations. There is a link between poor balance and scoliosis, so this is a vital test.

Scoliometer evaluation — This non-x-ray tool is used to approximate curve flexibility, size and location.

Spinal motion and static palpation — The doctor will move the spine gently to locate areas of inflammation and muscle tightness and to clarify location of restricted spinal segments.

Spinal cord tension testing — By determining the patient's flexibility and spinal cord length, the scoliosis specialist can prescribe appropriate stretching protocols. A shortened or tethered spinal cord can be an underlying cause of scoliosis progression.

Foot evaluation — A computerized foot scanner may be used to identify and analyze excessive rolling of the foot (pronation or supination).

Pain scales — A questionnaire is used to analyze pain patterns. This before-and-after evaluation tool will help clarify symptomatic recovery.

Vitals — Vital data, including weight, blood pressure and a very precise measurement of height are recorded. It is important to monitor height to see if a patient is growing or decreasing in height.

Your scoliosis specialist will use this evaluation data to determine the best treatment plan to reduce or correct your scoliosis.

More About X-ray Safety

The amount of x-ray exposure the patient receives from x-ray evaluation is always a concern to both doctor and patient. This concern must be weighed against the importance of knowledge gained from the examination.

As humans we are continuously bombarded by x-rays coming from natural sources. This radiation comes from outer space, the sun, the interior of the earth, radon gas and other natural sources. The amount of radiation we get from natural sources varies depending on the elevation at which we live and through our employment (think of an airplane crew). Comparative study results show that the radiation from typical scoliosis x-rays is similar to a small fraction of the annual exposure from natural sources.[33]

By using available x-ray-limiting technologies such as high-frequency x-ray generators, digital capture, smaller film sizes, lead and aluminum foil shielding, and x-ray-limiting settings on the machine, x-ray studies can be much safer and will expose the patient to significantly less radiation than standard full-spine films using conventional radiology.

New technologies have been developed to reduce radiation even further; however, at the time of the writing of this book, they are not deemed suitable for scoliosis evaluation except in extraordinary situations. A standing MRI allows for weight-bearing evaluation of scoliosis with zero radiation, but because of its high cost per evaluation, long scan time (*3-4 minutes during which the patient must hold perfectly still… very difficult, especially for a child*), and lack of standing MRI machines, this technology is not commonly used.

An ultra-low x-ray system called "the EOS," or slit scan technology, has similar limitations because the scan takes a long time. Raster stereography and Moire technology (also marketed as InSpeck, ISIS, Quantec and Frometric, which are based on the distortion which occurs when a grid of light

---

33 Pace, Nicola, Leonardo Ricci, and Stefano Negrini. "A Comparison Approach to Explain Risks Related to X-ray Imaging for Scoliosis, 2012 SOSORT Award Winner." *Scoliosis* 8.11 (2013): 7161-8. 19 Apr. 2016

is projected onto the back of the patient) hold great promise in analyzing scoliosis, but are not accurate enough to completely eliminate x-rays. Further research is needed in analyzing larger or obese patients and those with neuromuscular disorders.[34]

Radiation Exposure

While techniques vary from machine to machine and center to center, it is preferable for your scoliosis specialist to take "spot" view x-rays of the spine which typically expose the patient to very little radiation. The 1 mSv (millisievert, a unit of measure) of radiation emitted during a spot x-ray registers an Additional Cancer Risk of 0.014378 percent, which is equal to 1 in 6955 chances. (*Said another way, there is a 99.985622 percent chance of having no effect on the patient!*)

The chart below gives some perspective on radiation dosages by comparing the amount of radiation from various sources.

Comparison Doses			
Natural Background	3.1 mSv/year	**Domestic Pilots**	2.2 mSv/year
Average U.S. Exposure	6.2 mSv/year	**7-hour airline flight**	0.02 mSv
Spot X-ray	0.10 mSv	**Chest CT**	7.0 mSv

Ease Your Concerns

If you have concerns about your child's exposure to radiation or the type of x-rays being taken, discuss them with your scoliosis specialist. Ask your scoliosis specialist to provide lead shielding.

---

34 Knott, Patrick et al. "SOSORT 2012 Consensus Paper: Reducing X-ray Exposure in Pediatric Patients with Scoliosis." *Scoliosis* 9.1 (2014): 1. 21 Apr. 2016

There is a lead "shawl" which patients can wear during the x-rays that helps protect uninvolved areas of the body from x-ray exposure. In addition, specific foil filters can be used whenever possible to protect the thyroid, eyes and breasts. An additional lead shielding is used to protect the testicles or ovaries and thyroid gland. In addition to shielding, there are specific machine settings that lower the effective dose.

Is the damage due to low-dose radiation from medical imaging studies overstated? According to a group of eminent radiation scientists who published an article on the subject in the *American Journal of Clinical Oncology 2015*, the answer is a very strong "YES"! Read further by Googling "The Birth of the Illegitimate Linear No-threshold Model — An Invalid Paradigm for Estimating Risk Following Low-dose Radiation Exposure."[35]

35 Siegel, JA. "The Birth of the Illegitimate Linear No-Threshold Model: An ..." 2015. 26 Apr. 2016 <http://www.ncbi.nlm.nih.gov/pubmed/26535990>

Chapter 13. How is a Scoliosis Measured?

"Who was Cobb, and What is the Cobb Angle?"

The **Cobb angle** was first described in 1948 by Dr. John R. Cobb, an American orthopedic surgeon, who used a unique technique to measure the angle of spinal curves. It is a measurement that evaluates scoliosis curves on a front-to-back x-ray of the spine. A variation of this procedure is also used to measure kyphosis and lordosis.[36]

"How Does Someone Determine the Cobb Angle?"

A curve is measured using the position of the **end/transitional vertebrae.** The **end vertebra** are the upper and lowermost vertebrae which are the least displaced from the midline and the most severely tilted.

A line is drawn along the **superior (top) endplate** of the **top end vertebra,** and a

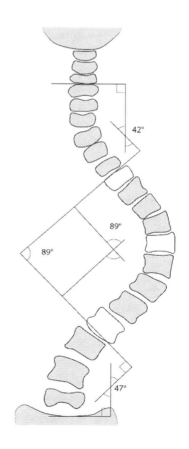

---

36 "Cobb angle — Wikipedia, the Free Encyclopedia." 2011. 31 Mar. 2016 <https://en.wikipedia.org/wiki/Cobb_angle>

second line is drawn along the **inferior (bottom) end plate** of the **bottom end vertebra**. The angle formed by these two lines (or the lines drawn perpendicular to them) is the Cobb angle.

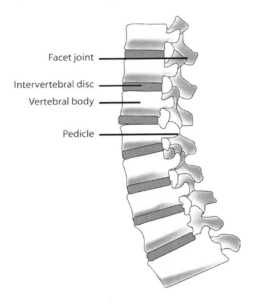

Facet joint

Intervertebral disc

Vertebral body

Pedicle

For S-shaped scoliosis, where there are two curves, the bottom end vertebra of the upper curve will represent the top end vertebra of the lower curve.

"What is the Significance of Cobb Angle?"

The Cobb angle is a measure of the curvature of the spine in degrees, which helps the doctor to determine what type of treatment is necessary. It is an imperfect way to evaluate the scoliosis because it is measuring a three-dimensional distortion in only two dimensions. The scoliosis is a rotation or twist in the spine and can only be accurately measured by high-tech, high-radiation computerized tomography (CT). Scoliosis specialists have all agreed to rely on the Cobb method measured on an x-ray because it's low-tech, and the analysis requires a low amount of radiation.

Typically, a Cobb angle of 10 is regarded as a minimum curve size to define scoliosis. Does that mean someone with a nine-degree curvature does not have scoliosis? Bizarrely, even though this is an arbitrary designation, in the medical world the answer is "yes!" For scoliosis curves between 10 – 20 degrees, orthopedic surgeons usually don't prescribe treatment, aside from regular check-ups. This is known as "watch and wait"...until the scoliosis becomes large enough to warrant bracing.

"What About a Custom-designed Exercise Program?"

Very few orthopedic surgeons have detailed knowledge of this approach, and therefore rarely recommend this active, low-risk and very effective treatment. Once the curve is 20-40 degrees, orthopedic surgeons generally prescribe one of several types of braces that are worn for 8-23 hours a day. Often times ineffective off-the-shelf braces are used with the idea they may slow progression until the child's spine has matured enough for the bones to hold metal screw implants. Design and construction of a modern over-corrective brace requires great expertise. Most orthopedic surgeons have only a cursory understanding of the complexities of customized, computer-designed scoliosis braces, so they rarely recommend using them.

"Why Do Cobb Angles Appear to Vary?"

Cobb angle is used worldwide to measure spinal abnormalities, particularly scoliosis. The Cobb angle measurement has become the gold standard of scoliosis evaluation and tracking and is endorsed by the Scoliosis Research Society.

The Adam's forward bend test is typically used to screen for scoliosis prior to puberty. If the test reveals signs of scoliosis, an x-ray is taken. If the x-ray indicates scoliosis, the Cobb angle is measured. However, because the Cobb angle reflects curvature only in a single plane, it fails to account for vertebral rotation, so it will not accurately demonstrate the severity of a three-dimensional spinal curvature.

Parents often ask, "Why does the Cobb angle calculation vary from doctor to doctor?" One reason is that patient placement affects measurement.

That's why it is important to have the scoliosis evaluated beyond simply knowing a Cobb angle. Scoliosis is a three-dimensional distortion of the spine, and the care plan must reflect that reality of which Cobb angle is only a small part.

Look at the following images of a coat hanger. They reflect what happens when Cobb angles differ, depending on when, where and how they are determined. Looking at the hanger from different angles yields very different angle calculations – yet it's the same hanger.

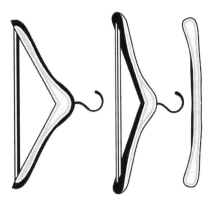

When a coat hanger is laying flat, the angle measures 60 degrees. If the coat hanger is rotated 90 degrees, the angle is zero. So when the hanger is in between, the angle measures 30 degrees. This demonstrates how a patient's Cobb angle changes in degrees simply due to even slight rotation while the x-ray is being taken. Therefore, a curve correction from 60 degrees to 30 degrees, as the result of treatment, will represent significantly more than a 50 percent correction of the 3-D scoliosis.

Time of day also impacts the measurement of the Cobb angle. Marc Beauchamp and his research team published a study in a 1993 edition of *Spine*, showing that the measurement of a back curve could vary by up to 5 degrees – and even as much as 10-20 degrees in rare cases.[37]

37 Beauchamp, Marc et al. "Diurnal Variation of Cobb Angle Measurement in Adolescent Idiopathic Scoliosis." *Spine* 18.12 (1993): 1581-1583. 18 Apr. 2016

> "Today the demands are for even higher standards in the quality of care, for greater flexibility and convenience in treatment times, and for more prevention through screening and health checks."
>
> - Lucy Powell

Chapter 14. School Screening For Scoliosis

"Is School Screening Valuable or a Huge Waste of Resources?"

There is a vast debate over whether to conduct scoliosis screenings in schools or not. The legislation varies from state to state in the United States. Here are both arguments:

If scoliosis screening in school is ineffective and unreliable and has no real impact on treatments or ultimate patient outcomes, why are more than half of our states still wasting time and money, pretending it has value?

On the other hand, people ask, "Are there effective early-stage treatment systems that can reduce scoliosis curve progression through exercise?" If yes, schools should be referring students to the scoliosis exercise specialists who offer early-stage treatment.

Since the 1960s, early detection of idiopathic scoliosis has become an expanding cause in the United States. Screening for scoliosis began in Aitkin, Minn., in 1963, and in 1973 the state of Minnesota enacted a statewide voluntary program.

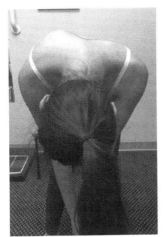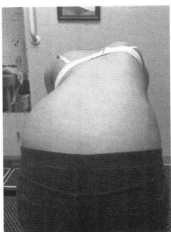

Adam's Forward Bend Test

The 2007 *Society on Scoliosis Orthopaedic and Rehabilitation Treatment* (SO-SORT) *Consensus Paper on School Screening for Scoliosis* that was discussed at the 4th International Conference on Conservative Management of Spinal Deformities specified that as of 2003, 21 states have legislated school screening. Of the remaining states, 11 recommend school screening without legislation, and the rest either have volunteer screenings or recommend not to conduct screening in the schools. National scoliosis school screening programs in Canada have been discontinued.[38]

In 2008, The American Academy of Orthopedic Surgeons (AAOS), Scoliosis Research Society (SRS), the Pediatric Orthopaedic Society of North America (POSNA), and the American Academy of Pediatrics (AAP) endorsed an information statement about screening for idiopathic scoliosis in adolescents. This statement does not recommend school screening programs, but does encourage the continuation of such programs where they currently exist and also states that they would not support any recommendations against screening.[39]

38 Grivas, TB. "SOSORT Consensus Paper: School Screening for ... — NCBI." 2007. 26 Apr. 2016 <http://www.ncbi.nlm.nih.gov/pmc/articles/PMC2228277/>

39 Labelle, H. "Screening for Adolescent Idiopathic Scoliosis: an ... — NCBI." 2013. 26 Apr. 2016 <http://www.ncbi.nlm.nih.gov/pmc/articles/PMC3835138/>

In 2013, after a review of research, the SRS International Task Force on Scoliosis screening, supported by the SRS Board of Directors, recommended screening girls twice at ages 10 and 12, and screening boys once at 13 or 14 years of age.

SCHOOL SCREENING IN U.S.

21 STATES LEGISLATED

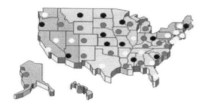

- 2002- VIRGINIA
- 1996-UTAH
- 1987-ARKANSAS
- 1985-TEXAS
- 1984-ALABAMA, INDIANA,
- 1983 - GEORGIA, NEVADA,
- 1982-CONNECTICUT, KENTUCKY, MARYLAND, PENNSYLVANIA
- 1981-MAINE, RHODE ISLAND
- 1980-CALIFORNIA, MASSACHUSETTS
- 1979-WASHINGTON, FLORIDA
- 1978-DELAWARE, NEW JERSEY, NEW YORK

- LEGISLATED
- RECOMMENDED
- NO RECOMMENDATION

AS OF 9/03

"Why Do Fewer Than Half of the U.S. States Mandate School Screening?"

Let's look at a few insights into this discrepancy. First, many programs have fallen out of favor because of "over-referral of adolescents with insignificant curves," which has been the source of much controversy.[40] There is a lack of research on the outcome of treatment as a result of early detection. In other words, if the bulk of scoliosis specialists aren't going to support custom-designed exercise-based home treatment for small curves, then why spend the money and time to find the small curve? This stance supports waiting – waiting until the mom or a friend notices a larger curve than a professional would see at a screening.

The Society on Scoliosis Orthopaedic and Rehabilitation Treatment (SO-SORT) states:

---

40 Reamy, Brian V, and Joseph B Slakey. "Adolescent Idiopathic Scoliosis: Review and Current Concepts." *American Family Physician* 64.1 (2001). Print.

> *"The policy not to screen because of lack of cost effectiveness is based on the obsolete assumption, derived from an early study that surgery is the only proven treatment option and the cited study does not justify scientifically this conclusion."*[41]

They suggest that intensive in-patient exercise programs can alter the scoliosis, and the rate of progression can be reduced significantly. Where conservative treatment is available at a high standard, the incidence of surgery can be significantly decreased. They reference articles that suggest school screening does reduce the number of surgically treated idiopathic scoliosis patients and emphasize the importance of recognizing the voluntary basis of the program in order to reduce the financial cost. They suggest that these findings support the idea that school screenings are a justified means of detecting mild and reversible spinal curvatures, so that they can be treated before they develop into spinal deformities with lifelong consequences and before they need surgical intervention.

SOSORT also addresses the dissimilarity and inconsistency of these programs as being one of the major hindrances of research:

> *"In the U.S.A., not all legislated screening programs are the same today. We can not take a broad-brush approach to whether or not a state has screening, but must look further at screening protocol details, including age and gender screened, screener education and support, scoliometer usage, reporting and follow-up methodologies etc, to evaluate the effectiveness of a program."*[42]

Typical screening tests are not very accurate and depend too much on the skill of the examiner. Examiners have a broad range of background from school nurse to gym instructor to specialist scoliosis clinician. Also, there is no national standard, which makes comparative research difficult and therefore hard to gauge what screening programs should be improved or

41 Grivas, TB. "SOSORT Consensus Paper: School Screening for ... — NCBI." 2007. 26 Apr. 2016 <http://www.ncbi.nlm.nih.gov/pmc/articles/PMC2228277/>

42 Grivas, TB. "SOSORT Consensus Paper: School Screening for ... — NCBI." 2007. 26 Apr. 2016 <http://www.ncbi.nlm.nih.gov/pmc/articles/PMC2228277/>

done away with. In addition, some schools have one nurse for every 700 students, and others have one nurse for 2000 students. Some school districts use health aides and volunteer parents to perform scoliosis screening.

A study published in 2011 that was conducted with 4,000 Norwegian children who were screened for scoliosis at age 12, found:

> "....acceptable sensitivity and specificity and low referral rates...age of 12 years only was not effective for detecting patients with indication for brace treatment. Screening should probably be initiated one year earlier for girls and one year later for boys, or be conducted more than once."[43]

This study used community nurses and physical therapists who completed educational courses to improve their knowledge of AIS, the Adam's forward bend test and measurement of rib arch using a scoliometer. This approach makes sense – a specialist team that travels to each school. The team would gain proficiency in scoliosis detection due to the vast numbers of children screened.

The goal of scoliosis screening is to detect it at an early stage when the deformity is likely to go unnoticed and when there is an opportunity for less invasive treatment. School screenings detect surface deformity. They don't attempt to predict which curves will progress and require treatment. Therefore, children with mild to moderate curves who are genetically predisposed to large curves might be diagnosed late, when curve progression has accelerated to beyond 30 degrees, making conservative management more challenging.

Universal screening supports early intervention and produces statistics that could aid research. Without screening, chances of early diagnosis are small as family doctors and pediatricians often don't check for scoliosis and, if they do they may only use the forward bend test which just shows a possible rib arch. The Adam's forward bend test (aka the "Adam's too-late test") is inadequate for evaluating early-stage scoliosis as it relies on rib cage dis-

43 Adobor, RD. "School Screening and Point Prevalence of ... — NCBI." 2011. 18 Apr. 2016 <http://www.ncbi.nlm.nih.gov/pmc/articles/PMC3213177/>

tortion, which only develops in thoracic spine curves above 20 degrees, neglecting lumbar spine curves.

Should screenings be conducted in schools? If so, what will ensure that they are consistently conducted with the same standards and protocols, but without increasing a challenged school budget?

II. WHAT CAUSES SCOLIOSIS?

Epigenetics and Scoliosis

Although considerable progress has been made in the past 25 years in understanding the underlying causes of adolescent scoliosis, there still is no agreed-upon theory of cause.

The main problem with determining a single cause appears to be that adolescent scoliosis does not result from one cause, but from multiple interacting factors along with a host of genetic predisposing factors.

To further complicate things, many researchers believe that there are two different and unique processes happening in scoliosis. First are the initiating processes, and second are the processes that cause curve progression. As the research unfolds there is increasing evidence of an underlying neurological disorder for adolescent scoliosis.

Epigenetics, a relatively new science, is analyzing factors from the environment, disease, aging, and even normal development that stimulates the genetic expression of scoliosis.

> "Scientists have found the gene for shyness. They would have found it years ago, but it was hiding behind a couple of other genes."
>
> — **Jonathan Katz**

Chapter 15. Scoliosis and Genetics

Scoliosis has been known to run in families. According to the University of Iowa Health Care department, "Hereditary and congenital irregularities have emerged as the most probable causes of scoliosis today." Based on population studies it is considered a single-gene disease with variable penetrance and heterogeneity.[44]

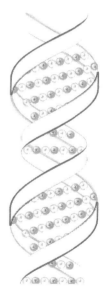

While genetics is believed to play a role in scoliosis, more than 80 percent of scoliosis cases are deemed idiopathic, meaning the source of the condition is unknown. Despite the vast amount of research, the cause of adolescent idiopathic scoliosis remains unknown. It is possible scoliosis is inherited the way other genetic traits are passed down from parent to child. This theory is greatly supported by the frequency with which scoliosis appears in families, co-occurring with parent, children and siblings. Studies have shown the incidence of scoliosis in these cases is in the 7–11 percent range. In contrast, the incidence in grandparent, grandchild, uncle, aunt, nephew, niece or half-sibling drops to less than 4 percent.

---

44 Tsiligiannis, T. "Pulmonary Function in Children with Idiopathic Scoliosis | Scoliosis and ..." 2012. 26 Apr. 2016 <http://scoliosisjournal.biomedcentral.com/articles/10.1186/1748-7161-7-7>

Factoid: *Actress Isabella Rossellini and her daughter, model Elettra Wiedemann, both have scoliosis.*

In 2007, Texas Scottish Rite Hospital for Children researchers identified the first gene – CHD7 – associated with idiopathic scoliosis. It was the result of a 10-year study led by Carol Wise, Ph.D., conducted at the Sarah M. and Charles E. Seay/Martha and Pat Beard Center for Excellence in Spine Research. In 2011, they identified two additional genes – CHL1 and DSCAM – which play a role in the neurological and spinal systems. These findings will allow for new hypotheses for the etiology of scoliosis and serve as a tool for further research.[45]

Alain Moreau, Ph.D., head of the molecular genetics lab for musculoskeletal diseases at the Ste-Justine University Hospital Centre, Montréal, Canada said in an interview:

> *"Most likely, scoliosis is not a purely genetic disease. Although genetic factors are important, a 'cross talk' between genetics and some environmental factors is evident. The nature of these environmental factors, however, is unclear. The underlying genetic defects may be present at birth, but because the clinical manifestations usually occur at adolescence or prepubescence, scoliotic deformities must be triggered by environmental factors, which also include hormonal changes associated with puberty.*
>
> *Increased levels of estrogen at puberty could explain why girls are more affected in number and severity than boys. Blood tests can now identify children at risk of developing scoliosis. We need to do more work on phenotype and trying to make sense of that and correlating it to genotype."[46]*

---

45 "Genetic Scoliosis Research — Texas Scottish Rite Hospital ..." 2013. 15 Apr. 2016 <http://www.tsrhc.org/genetic-scoliosis-research>

46 "Gene CHD7 Linked with Scoliosis [Archive] — National ..." 2009. 15 Apr. 2016 <http://www.scoliosis.org/forum/archive/index.php/t-8938.html>

So while genes may play a key role, like other genetic conditions, environmental factors may influence or even bring out this genetic predisposition. More genetic research and discoveries will fuel better understanding of the causes of scoliosis – specifically idiopathic scoliosis. Genetic research may provide the answer for what causes scoliosis, and it also may lead to improved preventive measures and treatment.

Chapter 16. Does Scoliosis Have Environmental Triggers?

It is believed that many people carry genes that trigger the development and/or progression of scoliosis. The genetics may or may not be "expressed," and the person may or may not develop scoliosis. Experts largely agree that a variety of genetic variations at the chromosomal level predispose a person to a condition like scoliosis. These genetic variants need to be activated or "turned on" by something.[47] That "something" has been studied intensely, according to scientific literature, and includes a wide variety of influencers. These "triggers" range from ONE OR EVEN SEVERAL of the following partial list:

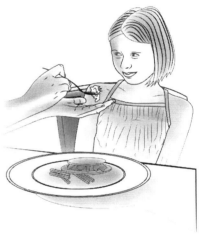

1. Abnormal development of the front of the spinal bones

2. Unsynchronized growth of the spine and the spinal cord

3. Instability in the spinal joints due to loss of normal curvature

4. Spinal disc disorders

---

47 Burwell, R Geoffrey et al. "Whither the Etiopathogenesis (and Scoliogeny) of Adolescent Idiopathic Scoliosis? Incorporating Presentations on Scoliogeny at the 2012 IRSSD and SRS Meetings." *Scoliosis* 8.1 (2013): 4. 21 Apr. 2016

5. Poor sensorimotor integration

6. Motor control disorder

7. Deformations of the spinal joints

8. Sensory integration disorder

9. Disorder of neurodevelopment

10. Defects of the shape of the inner ear

11. Defects in specific hormone receptors

12. Protein signaling defects

13. Maternal age at birth

14. Infants using heated indoor swimming pools

15. Body composition imbalances like obesity

16. Exposure to specific bacteria (mycobacteria)

17. Metabolism disorders including abnormalities of:

    a. Platelet calmodulin

    b. Melatonin

    c. Melatonin signaling defect

    d. Osteopontin

    e. Oestrogens

    f. Leptin

    g. Bone calcium (osteopenia)

18. Biomechanical misalignments of the spine and pelvis

19. Balance disorders

20. Body spatial disorientation

21. Trauma

22. Postural stress (e.g. heavy school bags)

23. Nutritional deficiencies and or excesses

Scoliosis and Nutrition

The impact that nutrition plays as an environmental influence on idiopathic scoliosis is not completely understood; however, more researchers are considering nutrition as a contributing factor in the manifestation of' scoliosis. While dietary changes are hardly the only care a scoliosis patient requires, let's take a look at what scientific studies are finding about the link between nutrition and scoliosis.

We know that poor nutrition can lead to many diseases, deformities and conditions. For example, though there is no single cause of spina bifida nor a known way to prevent it entirely, folic acid taken before and during pregnancy has been shown to reduce its incidence. Rickets, the most common childhood disease in developing countries, is bone softening attributed to a deficiency or impaired metabolism of vitamin D, phosphorus or calcium, potentially leading to fractures and deformity. Though it can occur in adults, the majority of cases occur in children suffering from severe malnutrition from famine or starvation during early childhood. Osteomalacia, a similar condition occurring in adults, is also generally due to a deficiency of vitamin D.

Could dietary deficiencies be the cause of idiopathic scoliosis, too? Researchers in one US study looked at articles from American and European journals, conference proceedings, and relevant research from 1955-1990 and found strong evidence (from animal studies) that poor nutrition could be a contributing factor in idiopathic scoliosis. While acknowledging limited human study data, they noted enough anecdotal evidence to warrant further investigation into a possible link between poor nutrition and the etiology of Idiopathic scoliosis.[48]

Other research shows a possible correlation between too much copper and scoliosis. Copper, an essential nutritional mineral is involved in energy production and the formation of red blood cells, bone and hemoglobin. It is also essential to nerve health, building and maintaining myelin, the insu-

---

48 Worthington, V. "Nutrition as an Environmental Factor in the Etiology of ... — NCBI." 1993. 26 Apr. 2016. <http://www.ncbi.nlm.nih.gov/pubmed/8492060>

lating sheath that surrounds nerve cells. Copper aids an enzyme involved in the production of collagen and elastin, two connective tissue proteins. Copper also works with zinc and vitamin C to form elastin. It's necessary for the development and the maintenance of skin, bones, blood vessels and joints, but can be problematic if elevated.[49]

Copper Function

A 2008 study from Czechia (Czech Republic) showed the changes of selenium, copper and zinc content in hair and serum of patients with idiopathic scoliosis. The patients studied were age 13 on average and had idiopathic scoliosis curves ranging between 12 and 82 degrees. The hair of these patients showed significantly increased zinc and copper (Cu) content and decreased selenium (Se) content when compared with the control group. The Cu/Se ratio in this group of patients was significantly higher due to a higher Cu value and a lower Se value in comparison with the controls. Also, compared with the controls, the serum selenium concentration in the group of scoliotic patients was significantly decreased.[50]

A 2002 study from Czechia on idiopathic scoliosis and concentrations of zinc, copper, selenium, albumin, and ceruloplasmin in blood and the activity of superoxide dismutase plasma found a significant decrease of selenium when compared with a control group. The same levels of significance were found for selenium levels corrected for albumin content.

In a group of patients with a curvature over 45 degrees (medically this size curve is often recommended for surgical intervention) the average plasma concentrations of selenium were significantly lower in comparison with a group of patients with a curvature below 45 degrees who were treated conservatively.

---

49 Burwell, RG. "Adolescent Idiopathic Scoliosis (AIS), Environment..." 2011. 25 Apr. 2016. <http://scoliosisjournal.biomedcentral.com/articles/10.1186/1748-7161-6-26>

50 Dastych, M. "Changes of Selenium, Copper, and Zinc Content in Hair and ..." 2008. <http://www.ncbi.nlm.nih.gov/pubmed/18404661> 25 Apr. 2016.

The decreased concentration of selenium in the blood plasma suggests possible negative effects on the process of synthesis and maturation of collagen affecting axial skeleton (i.e, skull, spine, ribs) stability.[51]

Just to show that there is no consensus on selenium, an article from China says the opposite, stating high selenium levels are linked as a risk factor for developing scoliosis!

Nearly 10,000 cases from three areas in China were included in this study. Each region had different selenium levels.

Researchers found high selenium levels significantly associated with AIS development, whereas low selenium levels had no significant correlation with AIS development. They also found that females in the high selenium group had larger curves than males. These results align with typical male/female presentation seen with idiopathic scoliosis.

This study confirmed that high selenium content was one of risk factors for idiopathic scoliosis. The authors of the study suggest that very high selenium levels may not cause scoliosis as the symptoms of selenium poisoning do not include scoliosis. However, a large number of animal experiments suggested that ingesting a certain amount of selenium would significantly boost body development. They suggest that the "growth-promoting effect of selenium" resulted in spinal overgrowth during the growth cycle and lead to scoliosis. But this hypothesis was still inconsistent with some phenomena during investigation. They did not find any height differences among the three areas and can't explain why males seem more susceptible to the effects of high selenium.[52]

As indicated at the beginning of this article, scoliosis is most likely caused by a genetic predisposition brought out by some external force. Some research suggests a link between nutrition and AIS, but this is probably an

51 Dastych, M. "Idiopathic Scoliosis and Concentrations of Zinc ... — NCBI." 2002. <http://www.ncbi.nlm.nih.gov/pubmed/12449234> 25 Apr. 2016.

52 Ji, X et al. "Change of Selenium in Environment and Risk of Adolescent Idiopathic Scoliosis: a Retrospective Cohort Study." *Eur Rev Med Pharmacol Sci* 17.18 (2013): 2499-503. 21 Apr. 2016.

effect of a genetic defect rather than a cause. Perhaps the gene(s) responsible for scoliosis are also responsible for the malabsorption/retention of certain nutrients in the scoliotic patient. In other words, it may not be that the patient has poor eating habits, but that they have a biological inability to store or remove certain nutrients in their body.

AIS is associated with whole organism metabolic phenomena, including lower body mass index, lower circulating leptin levels and other systemic disorders (those which affect multiple parts or the whole body).[53]

---

53 Burwell, RG. "Scoliogeny of Adolescent Idiopathic Scoliosis: Inviting ..." 2013. 25 Apr. 2016. <http://scoliosisjournal.biomedcentral.com/articles/10.1186/1748-7161-8-8>

> *"All too often when liberals cite statistics, they forget the statisticians' warning that correlation is not causation."*
>
> **– Thomas Sowell**

Chapter 17. Are a Child's Thinness and Scoliosis Linked?

Though we don't completely understand why, certain common characteristics exist among adolescents with scoliosis — one of the common characteristics is having a small build or low weight. This inexplicable commonality has led to newer research that focuses on body mass and its possible connection to adolescent idiopathic scoliosis.

A 2012 study conducted in Spain researched body composition in relation to adolescent idiopathic scoliosis. Researchers used body mass index (BMI) and body shape in girls with AIS and compared them with non-scoliotic girls of the same age.

> *"AIS and anorexia nervosa (AN) make their debut during adolescence and both may be associated with an alteration of their subjective physical perception. Some authors propose a link between AIS and AN, supported both by an alteration of physical perception and lower BMI."*[54]

---

54 Ramírez, M. "Body Composition in Adolescent Idiopathic Scoliosis — NCBI." 2013. 26 Apr. 2016. <http://www.ncbi.nlm.nih.gov/pmc/articles/PMC3555626/>

BMI CHART (Body Mass Index) A measure of body fat based on height and weight.	
BMI less than 18.5	Underweight
BMI 18.5 — 24.9	Healthy weight
BMI 25.0 — 29.9	Overweight
BMI 30.0 or more	Obese

A study population of more than 5,000 patients that was published by Kyle et al. was chosen as a control (Group 1). Another control group (Group 2) of healthy volunteers matched by sex and age was selected among a school-age and university population in Barcelona, Spain. Twenty seven female AIS surgery candidates were studied (average age: 17 years/ average BMI: 18.9). A significant difference in BMI between AIS and Group 1 was observed (21.0 vs.18.9; fat-free mass (FFM = 42.6 vs. 38.9) and fat mass (FM = 15.6 vs.13.7). Significant differences in BMI (22.13 vs. 18.9), fat mass index (FMi = 7.17 vs. 4.97) and fat-free mass index (FFMi = 14.95 vs. 13.09) between AIS and Group 2 also were seen. They found BMI, FFMi and FMi were all lower in the AIS participants than in the general population included in the study.[55]

Could this mean a link between eating disorders and scoliosis? A later study in 2013 would disagree. It stated: "A recent study suggests a correlation between idiopathic scoliosis in adolescence and eating disorders. However, this does not correspond with our clinical experience in the same population."[56]

They did find BMI to be slightly lower for scoliosis patients, as it is reported in most literature on scoliosis. However, by using the EAT-26 questionnaire (recognized among the most valid questionnaires for eating disorders and widely applied in various countries), researchers found a lower incidence of

---

55 Ramírez, Manuel et al. "Body Composition in Adolescent Idiopathic Scoliosis." *European Spine Journal* 22.2 (2013): 324-329. Print.

56 Zaina, F. "Adolescent Idiopathic Scoliosis and Eating Disorders: is ..." 2013. <http://www.ncbi.nlm.nih.gov/pubmed/23357674> 25 Apr. 2016.

eating disorders in female scoliosis patients than in the general population. They used both their own controls and Italian reference values.[57]

A 2014 Korean study expanded on the connection between AIS progression and longitudinal growth during puberty seen in female AIS patients, to a discussion including male AIS patients. The study compared height, weight and BMI of young males with normal spinal curves with male AIS subjects. They also compared patients by curve severity. They found Korean AIS males had significantly different somatometric results — specifically, greater height and lower weight. Furthermore, body weight was significantly lower in the severe group than in the moderate group. This shows abnormal growth is observed in male AIS and that body weight is correlated with AIS severity.[58]

Another 2014 study looked at the prevalence of adolescent spinal deformities according to severity, as well as their possible link to BMI and height. Subjects' curves were classified as mild, intermediate or severe, according to standing x-ray measurements. The study included 829,791 consecutive subjects of whom 103,249 were diagnosed with spinal deformities. The instance of spinal deformities was significantly greater among the underweight male and female patients. Increased BMI had a protective effect for developing spinal deformities. The odds for severe spinal deformities were greater compared with mild spinal deformities in the underweight groups. The risk for developing spinal deformities increased significantly with height for both genders.[59]

Looking over these studies, you will conclude — as I have — that results are conflicting. Do scoliosis kids have it because they are thin, or are they thin because they have scoliosis? We need more research!

---

57 Zaina, F. "Adolescent Idiopathic Scoliosis and Eating Disorders: is ..." 2013. <http://www.ncbi.nlm.nih.gov/pubmed/23357674> 25 Apr. 2016.

58 Oh, CH. "A Comparison of the Somatometric Measurements of ... — NCBI." 2014. 26 Apr. 2016. <http://www.ncbi.nlm.nih.gov/pubmed/23511644>

59 Hershkovich, O. "Association Between Body Mass Index, Body Height ... — NCBI." 2014. 26 Apr. 2016. <http://www.ncbi.nlm.nih.gov/pubmed/24332597>

Chapter 18. The Puberty-Scoliosis Connection

Scoliosis in adolescence is one of the most frequent forms of postural distortion, and it occurs most frequently in pubescent girls.

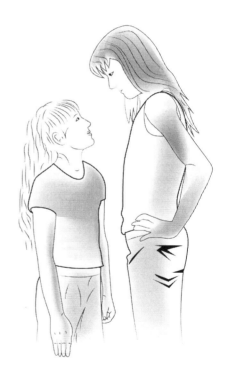

Studies suggest that one of the catalysts for this manifestation of AIS may involve a significant disorder of estrogens, the hormones that trigger the onset of puberty.

One such study tested concentrations of FSH, LH, estrogens, progesterone, osteocalcin, RANKL and the activity of alkaline phosphatase (AP) in prepubescent and postpubescent scoliotic girls and compared them to samples taken from non-scoliotic pre- and postpubescent girls

...Okay, dear reader! Hang on here! This is going to get a little more technical, so stick with me or feel free to skip to the end of this chapter for my summary on hormones and scoliosis.

Before we discuss the details of the research, the following chart will give a breakdown of what was tested, how each hormone functions within the body, and their levels in pre- and postpubescent scoliotic girls when compared to non-scoliotic peers.

What was Tested

This chart illustrates the range and normal function of female hormones. The chart then compares the levels of each hormone in girls with scoliosis before and after they have begun their menstrual cycle compared to a group of girls without scoliosis.

	Function	Premenarcheal Scoliotic Girls	Postmenarcheal Scoliotic Girls
FSH (Follicle-stimulating hormone)	Regulates the development, growth, pubertal maturation and reproductive processes of the body. FSH and luteinizing hormone (LH) act synergistically in reproduction.	Lower	Lower
LH (Luteinizing hormone)	Produced by gonadotroph cells in the anterior pituitary gland. In females, an acute rise of LH triggers ovulation. Luteinizing hormone and follicle-stimulating hormone levels rise and fall together during the monthly menstrual cycle.	Lower	Lower
Estradiol (One of several natural estrogens)	Predominant estrogen during reproductive years. Regulates menstrual cycles	Lower	Lower

	Function	Preme-narcheal Scoliotic Girls	Postme-narcheal Scoliotic Girls
Estrone (One of several natural estrogens)	Least abundant of the three estrogens, Estrone converts to estrone sulfate, a long-lived derivative. Estrone sulfate acts as a reservoir that can be converted as needed to the more active estradiol. It is the predominant estrogen in postmenopausal women.	Similar to control	Slightly lower
Estriol (One of several natural estrogens)	Abundant primarily during pregnancy	Similar to control	Same
Progesterone	Involved in the menstrual cycle, pregnancy, and embryogenesis. Progesterone levels are relatively low during the preovulatory phase of the menstrual cycle, rise after ovulation, and are elevated during the luteal phase. Progesterone levels are relatively low in children and postmenopausal women.	Higher	Lower
AP (Alkaline phosphatase)	A byproduct of osteoblast activity, AP increases if there is active bone formation occurring. Levels are significantly higher in children and pregnant women.	Higher	Higher
Osteocalcin	Secreted solely by osteoblasts and thought to play a role in the body's metabolic regulation and is pro-osteoblastic, or bone-building.	Higher	Higher

	Function	Preme-narcheal Scoliotic Girls	Postme-narcheal Scoliotic Girls
RANKL (Receptor activator of nuclear factor kappa-B ligand)	Through the binding of RANKL, osteoclasts and osteoblasts play a vital role in normal bone remodeling. Overproduction of RANKL is implicated in a variety of degenerative bone diseases (e.g. rheumatoid arthritis and psoriatic arthritis).	Higher	Higher

"What Were the Findings?"

In **PREmenarcheal scoliotic girls**, the levels of FSH, LH and estradiol were lower; the levels of progesterone were higher; and the concentrations of estrone and estriol were similar compared to girls without scoliosis. Higher levels of RANKL, osteocalcin and AP were observed in premenarcheal adolescents with AIS compared with non-scoliosis.

In **POSTmenarcheal scoliotic girls,** the levels of FSH, LH, estradiol and progesterone were lower, estrone were slightly lower, and estriol did not differ compared with the control group. Significantly higher levels of RANKL, osteocalcin and AP were observed in postmenarcheal scoliotic adolescents compared with controls.

They suggest that such findings can be explained by delayed puberty. The average age of girls with AIS was higher in both pre- and postmenarcheal groups compared to the groups without AIS.

> *"There is an interdependence between the concentration of estradiol and development of scoliosis. Determination of estradiol may have diagnostic value in the screening of spinal pathologies associated with AIS."*[60]

---

60 Kulis, Aleksandra et al. "Participation of Sex Hormones in Multifactorial Pathogenesis of Adolescent Idiopathic Scoliosis." *International Orthopaedics* 39.6 (2015): 1227-1236. 19 Apr. 2016.

As the authors state, there is already plenty of research that supports a multifactorial cause of scoliosis and (as we've previously mentioned) the involvement of genetic and epigenetic predispositions and the influence of hormonal factors are also widely accepted. Scoliosis is assumed to be associated with a sex-linked predominant gene with incomplete penetrance (meaning that symptoms are not always present in individuals who have the genetic mutation) and variable expression (meaning variations in type and severity of a genetic disorder can exist between individuals with the same genetic mutation, even within the same family).

There are **twice as many girls than boys with Cobb angles greater than 10 degrees and eight times as many with Cobb angles greater than 30 degrees.** Are hormones the only reason AIS occurs more frequently in girls than boys? The study goes on to reference another study from 2012 that explains how adolescent idiopathic scoliosis occurs 2-10 times more frequently in females than in males. This observation is postulated to be due to the **Carter effect.** (Males are more likely to transmit the disease to their children, but not have AIS themselves.) In this situation males would need to inherit a greater number of susceptibility genes compared to females to develop AIS and would also be more likely to transmit the disease to their children and to have siblings with AIS. In the families they tested, AIS was lowest in sons of affected mothers (36%) and highest in daughters of affected fathers (85%). Affected fathers transmitted AIS to 80 percent of the children in the test, whereas affected mothers transmitted it to 56 percent. Siblings of affected males also had a significantly higher prevalence of AIS (55%) compared with siblings of affected females (45%). They state that the presence of the Carter effect supports the multifactorial threshold model of inheritance in AIS.[61]

"What Role Might Estrogen Have in Scoliosis Formation?"

It is believed that AIS develops in two stages: **1)** initial functional impairment of osteoblasts and osteoclasts (which control the amount of bone tissue: osteoblasts form bone, osteoclasts repair/remodel bone), and **2)** the stage of actual spinal deformation. However, the reason is still unknown.

---

61 Kruse, LM. "Polygenic Threshold Model with Sex Dimorphism in ... — NCBI." 2012. 26 Apr. 2016. <http://www.ncbi.nlm.nih.gov/pubmed/22992817>

Estrogens have a modifying influence on bone growth and remodeling, and control changes in the structure of cancellous bones (spongy bone). The authors are not suggesting that estrogens cause AIS, but that due to their function, they may affect progression. Estrogen deficiency is associated with increased bone turnover, increased osteoclast activity and increased osteoblast activity. Estrogens also modulate the activity of the melatonin receptor and inhibit the synthesis of melatonin. They interact with other hormones and biochemical factors, such as calcium-binding protein calmodulin, as well as with other proteins controlling muscle contractility.

> *"Understanding the role of estrogens seems vital for explaining the evolution of AIS associated with skeletal growth..."*[62]

62 Kulis, Aleksandra et al. "Participation of Sex Hormones in Multifactorial Pathogenesis of Adolescent Idiopathic Scoliosis." *International Orthopaedics* 39.6 (2015): 1227-1236. 19 Apr. 2016.

Chapter 19. Can Baby Walkers 'Turn On' Scoliosis Gene?

This chapter is based on the writings and research of Dr. Fred Barge, chiropractor.

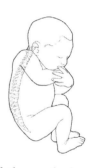

Babies begin life with C-shaped spinal curves. This is referred to as the primary curve. The secondary spinal curves are not yet developed, as is evident in a newborn's inability to hold its head up.

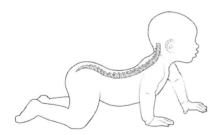

The secondary curve of the neck develops when the baby is placed on its stomach during tummy time, and he starts to strengthen neck muscles by lifting his head. This develops the cervical lordotic curve, a normal neck curve.

Tummy time allows babies to develop their secondary neck curves and prepares their spinal muscles for upright posture. To develop the secondary lumbar

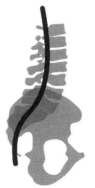

Lordotic
Lumbar Spine

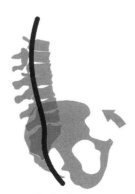

Kyphotic
Lumbar Spine

lordotic curve in the lower back, babies "creep" or push themselves around on their tummies. The first few months are crucial in the baby's spine development.

There are many products on the market (many of which have been around for years) that are used to keep babies entertained and safe. However, most of these devices inhibit the development of secondary curves. Baby walkers, swings and door frame jumpers hold the spine in a "C" position and inhibit development of secondary spinal curves. Some of these products, like the walker, even allow infants to stand on their feet with erect posture before their spine and pelvis are developed and before their spines are ready to support the weight of standing upright.

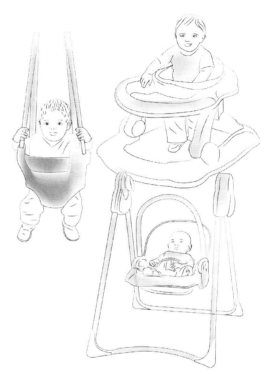

Use of these devices can lead to early walking. Because the lumbar spine has not formed its anterior curve yet, early walking can also lead to a flattening of the lower back called kyphosis.

Low-back kyphosis puts undue pressure on spinal discs and can cause disc wedging and vertebral misalignments called "subluxations."[63] The spine can shift to one side and then the other, to compensate. This type of spinal instability can trigger the body to develop a mild curvature. If conditions are right, this can then develop into a full blown scoliosis. Since the child's spine

---

63 "Chiropractic — Mission of the World Chiropractic Alliance." 20 Apr. 2016 <http://www.worldchiropracticalliance.org/>

is still developing, they will adapt to this curve, unless the subluxations and disc wedging are corrected before puberty.

While most of these products are useful for busy parents, time spent in them should be limited and interchanged with more "tummy time" and creeping and crawling later on. These are the best positions for babies to be in when active. Many products place emphasis on their ability to allow babies to walk sooner, but because infants may not be physically ready to do so, this can be an unfavorable encouragement. By allowing infants to spend time on their stomachs, they gradually are able to reach milestones like creeping, crawling, cruising and walking – when their bodies are biomechanically prepared to do so.

So...do baby swings, jumpers and walkers cause scoliosis? As we've mentioned, current thinking is that cases of AIS are caused by a genetic predisposition for scoliosis that gets triggered. The use of these products in infancy is one possible trigger for scoliosis expression. In all other cases, excessive use of these products still has damaging effects. While it will not result in scoliosis for all, it may still lead to improper development of some spine contours which can lead to a general spinal weakening in adulthood and a flattening of the lower back.[64]

---

64 Jackson, R. "The Classic: The Cervical Syndrome — NCBI — National ..." 2010. 26 Apr. 2016. <http://www.ncbi.nlm.nih.gov/pmc/articles/PMC2881998/>

Chapter 20. How Do Normal Daily Activities Affect Scoliosis?

Normal Daily Activities are also known as "Activities of Daily Living" (ADLs). These are the activities that people do routinely everyday.

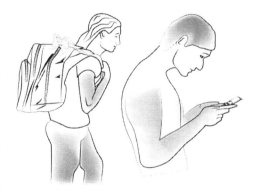

We all know that improper posture, both standing and seated, is bad for the joints and especially bad for the back, but could it be worse for scoliosis? Research suggests that while poor posture can not "cause" scoliosis, poor posture can exacerbate scoliosis. Specifically, increased time spent in a seated position – an improper seated position – can lead to asymmetry of the spine and scoliosis.

A study published in 2014 examined the effects of seated position on children age 11 to 13. Researchers found that sitting caused a flattening of the normal and healthy curve of the middle back.[65]

Slouching! This has been suggested as a risk factor leading to the expression of scoliosis. This may not come as a shock, given the amount of time chil-

---

65 Drza-Grabiec, J. "Effects of the Sitting Position on the Body Posture of ... — NCBI." 2015. 26 Apr. 2016. <http://www.ncbi.nlm.nih.gov/pubmed/24962297>

dren and adults sit at school, in a car or bus, in front of a computer playing video games. As technology advances and life becomes more automated, we are able to stay seated for longer periods.

> *"Current evidence suggests that North American children and youth spend between 40 percent and 60 percent of their waking hours engaging in sedentary pursuits."*[66]

"Is Sitting the Only Issue? What About Other Activities?"

Sitting is an issue, but let's look at a little closer at other activities common to daily living.

Ergonomics is the scientific study of how people interact with their environment in order to eliminates injuries or disorders that can develop from repetitive movements, bad posture and overuse of muscles. Businesses capitalize on findings by designing ergonomic furniture and products to make movements easier and to prevent injury.[67]

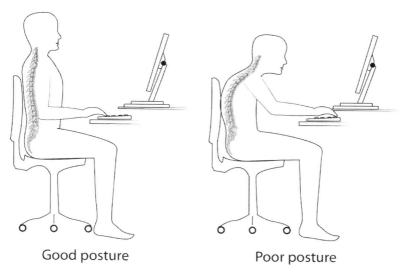

Good posture   Poor posture

66 Saunders, Travis J, Jean-Philippe Chaput, and Mark S Tremblay. "Sedentary Behaviour as an Emerging Risk Factor for Cardiometabolic Diseases in Children and Youth." *Canadian Journal of Diabetes* 38.1 (2014): 53-61. Print.

67 "CDC — Ergonomics and Musculoskeletal Disorders — NIOSH ..." 2003. 20 Apr. 2016 <http://www.cdc.gov/niosh/topics/ergonomics/>

Improvements to health and posture, however, are not necessarily linked to spending money. Modifications to **activities of daily living** (ADLs) at home, school or work can make a huge difference in posture.

How you sit in a chair matters, particularly if you are in it for hours on end. How you carry a tote or purse affects posture, too.

Have you ever noticed that it's easier to carry a purse or messenger bag on one shoulder than on the other side? Why is that?

Does carrying a heavy purse or backpack cause permanent damage? What kind of damage could it cause?

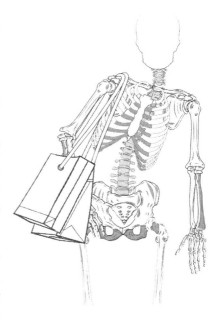

The adjacent image depicts the effect of carrying a bag on one shoulder. Notice how the body naturally leans in the opposite direction to compensate for the added weight.

Now imagine that this person already has a spinal curvature toward the right. It is possible to modify how you carry your backpack, purse or groceries to help manage scoliosis.

Malaysian researchers found that a single session of ergonomic intervention showed significant improvements in the seated posture of children. Reduction of schoolbag weight helped, too.

They recommended early intervention, ergonomics education programs for children aged 8 and 11 years to reduce musculoskeletal damage and pain.[68]

---

68 Syazwan, A. "Poor Sitting Posture and a Heavy Schoolbag as ... — NCBI." 2011. 26 Apr. 2016. <http://www.ncbi.nlm.nih.gov/pubmed/22003301>

Patients are always asking me what they can do outside of their scoliosis treatment program to help reduce pain or encourage their curve reduction. I have developed a program to assess what comprises patients' daily activities and what modifications can benefit their spinal curvatures. I have presented this at an advanced scoliosis conference, and now many scoliosis clinicians are helping their patients with simple modifications to their normal everyday activities.

As a follow-up to this book, I will be writing a self-help book for children and adults with scoliosis.

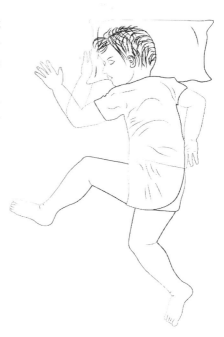

The method of tweaking activities of daily living will be explored in detail there. The method is called Active Self Correction and is the common link amongst all the European scoliosis specific exercise programs.

> "We know from our clinical experience in the practice of medicine that in diagnosis, prognosis, and treatment, the individual and his background of heredity are just as important, if not more so, as the disease itself."
>
> – Paul Dudley White

III. SCOLIOSIS TREATMENT

> "Those who do not remember the past are condemned to repeat it."
>
> – **George Santayana**

Chapter 21. Bizarre Historical Scoliosis Treatments

The existence of scoliosis in humans is likely as old as the existence of man. There is a long history of its presentation from King Tutankhamun to Hippocrates. Because of this, there is a vast and fascinating history of both the condition and its treatment. Interestingly, many of the bygone forms of treatment are very similar to today's treatments.

An article published in the 2009 *Scoliosis Journal* details the history of spinal deformities and their treatment. In Ancient Greece "medicine" was practiced at Asclepions, temples dedicated to Aesculapius, the god of health. A priest-physician conducted treatments such as hydrotherapy, physiotherapy, hygienic rule, diet, drug therapies and minor surgical procedures. (Figure 1)[69]

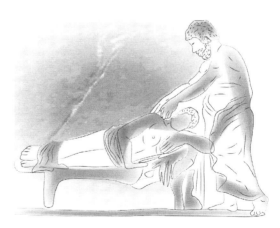

Figure 1. Aesculapius, the god of health, examines a patient

69 Vasiliadis, ES. "Historical Overview of Spinal Deformities in Ancient Greece ..." 2009. 26 Apr. 2016. <http://scoliosisjournal.biomedcentral.com/articles/10.1186/1748-7161-4-6>

The authors suggest that such practices were most likely also used to treat spinal deformities.

Hippocrates (460-370 B.C.) recommended diet and extension for the treatment of scoliosis. During the time of Hippocrates, spinal manipulation was widely used as a treatment for scoliosis; however, he was the first to invent devices based on principles of stretching and lengthening the spine, as well as how to apply corrective pressure to straighten spinal curvatures. Hippocratic books do not contain illustrations of these techniques but Apollonius of Kitium (first century B.C.) wrote of Hippocrates techniques in *On Articulations,* and illustrations were found in a Florentine surgical manuscript (*Laurentianus 74. 7*, ninth century) (Figures 2, 3 and 5).

Hippocratic Ladder

The Hippocratic ladder was developed to reduce spinal curvatures. To achieve reduction, the patient was shaken while tied on a ladder – in an erect position if the rib arch was near the neck or with the head downward if the rib arch was at a lower level. Body weight pulled and straightened the spine. Hippocrates described the board as the most efficient method for the correction of spinal deformities because the physician could easily control the forces exercised on the spine and those forces were exerted naturally (Figure 2).

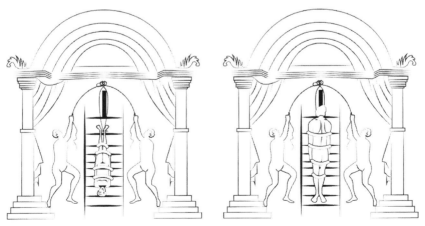

Figure 2. Hippocratic Ladder.

Hippocratic Board

The Hippocratic Board is another device to manage spinal curvatures. Simultaneous traction of the spine and the manual application of focal pressure over the kyphotic area was recommended:

> *"But the physicians, or some person who is strong, and not uninstructed, should apply the palm of the hand to the hump, and then, having laid the other hand upon the former, he should make pressure, attending whether this force should be applied directly downward, or toward the head, or toward the hips ... and there is nothing to prevent a person from placing a foot on the hump, and supporting his weight on it, and making gentle pressure; one of the men who is practiced in the palestra*[70] would be a proper person for doing this in a suitable manner." (Figures 3 and 4).*

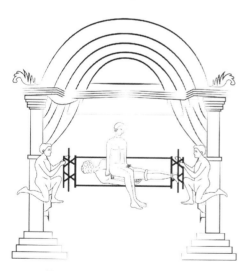

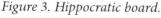

Figure 3. Hippocratic board.

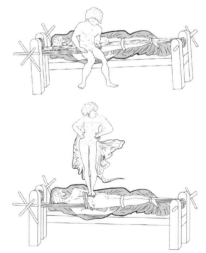

Figure 4. Correction of
spinal deformity with the
Hippocratic board.

---

70 * A public place in ancient Greece for training and practice in wrestling and other athletics.

For patients requiring stronger forces, Hippocrates recommended:

> "*The apparatus for forcible reduction should be arranged as follows. One may fix in the ground a strong broad plank having in it a transverse groove. Or, instead of the plank, one may cut a transverse groove in a wall, a cubit above the ground, or as may be convenient. Then place a sort of quadrangular oak board parallel with the wall and far enough from it that one may pass between if necessary; and spread cloaks on the board, or something that shall be soft, but not very yielding....*" *(Figure 6)*

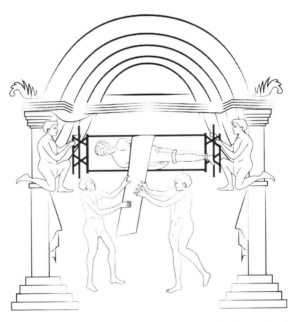

Figure 6. Hippocratic board used with a plank on the hump.

> "*...A soft band, sufficiently broad and long, composed of two strands, should be applied at its middle to the middle of the chest, and passed twice round it as near as possible to the armpits; then let what remains of the (two) bands be passed round the shoulders at each side, and the ends be attached to a pestle-shaped pole, adjusting their length to that of the underlying board against which the pestle-shaped pole is put, using it as a fulcrum to make extension.*" *(Figure 7).*

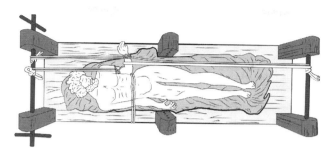

Figure 7. Use of straps and bands on the Hippocratic board.

Oribasius (325-400 A.D.), a Byzantine physician, modified the Hippocratic board by adding a bar. He used it for gradual reduction of both spinal traumas and deformities. (Figure 8).

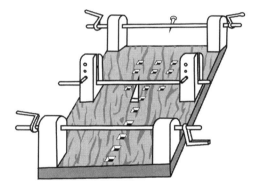

Figure 8. A third bar was added to the Hippocratic board.

Hippocratic Scamnum

The third device for the management of spinal deformities was the Hippocratic scamnum (Figure 9):

> *"But the most powerful of the mechanical means is this; if the hole in the wall, or in the piece of wood fastened into the ground, be made as much below the man's back as may be judged proper, and if a board, made of lime-tree, or any wood, and not too narrow, be put into the hole, then a rag, folded several times or a small leather cushion,*

should be laid on the hump ... when matters are thus adjusted, one
person, or two if necessary, must press down at the end of the board,
while others at the same time make extension and counter-extension
along the body, as formerly described."

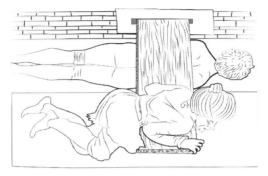

Figure 9. The Hippocratic scamnum.

Galen (129–216 A.D.) recommended the use of the Hippocratic
board (Figure 10) for traumatic deformities and the Hippocratic ladder for kyphotic deformities, although he expressed his doubts on
the effectiveness of this technique.

Paulus of Aegina (625–690 A.D.)
lived during the Byzantine period,
but is still considered the last physician of Greek antiquity. He used

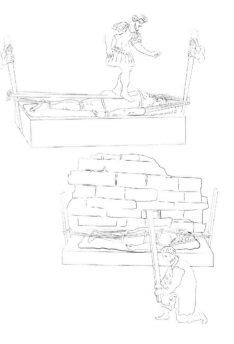

Figure 10. Galen's devices were
similar to the Hippocratic board
and scamnum.

the Hippocratic board for management of spinal deformities and also emphasized it in the use of orthoses in spinal trauma and deformities.[71]

Controversy surrounded the next methods I am going to describe. These protocols were used in France as early as 1820, documents show.

At the time, surgeons were using powerful mechanical means to perform traction on the spinal column to correct deformity, which in some cases led to paralysis. The Royal Academy of Medicine was involved and certain practices were discredited.

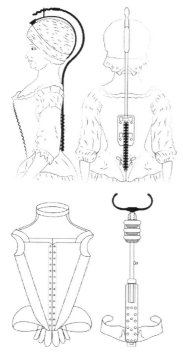

Figure 11. Extension chair
by Levacher.

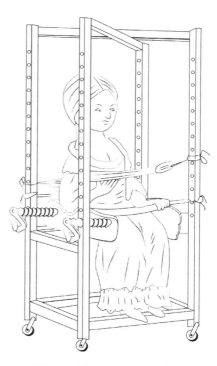

Figure 12. Minerva jacket
by Levacher.

71 Vasiliadis, ES. "Historical Overview of Spinal Deformities in Ancient Greece ..." 2009. 26 Apr. 2016. <http://scoliosisjournal.biomedcentral.com/articles/10.1186/1748-7161-4-6>

Surgeons set up a research society to monitor the complications. As recently as 1975, the
research society reported an
incidence of paralysis of 0.72
percent (57 cases!) in a sample
of 7885 patients. There were
many causes, but excessive
traction on the spinal column
most definitely caused pre-
ventable paralysis. The transmitted force on the spinal cord
and the nerve roots would
have been tremendous once
surgeons cut stabilizing ligaments. Paralysis also resulted
when forcible traction was applied by halo – even without
dividing the ligaments.

In 1764, Francois Guillaume
Levacher de la Feutrie introduced the first mechanical

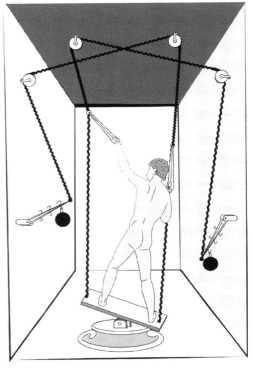

*Figure 13. Balançoire Othopédique
by Pravaz.*

bed in France. The bed was designed to "push on the bumps" in an attempt
to cure rickets. It only was used on children because of their soft adaptable
bones. It would have been used periodically for up to two weeks at a time,
applying gentle pressure. The bed did not exert traction on both extremities
of the body, therefore avoiding adverse effects (Figures 11 and 12).

Charles Gabriel Pravaz (1791-1853) believed scoliosis resulted from une-
qual growth or activity. His extension equipment allowed patients to remain
in an upright position as he was a critic of the previously designed hori-
zontal beds. He emphasized the importance for patients to self-adjust the
traction. Pravaz used gentle traction therapy for no more than two hours a
day with no adverse effects (Figure 13).

In the 1820s, Charles-Auguste Maisonabe introduced his version of the mechanical bed, which used weights attached to straps or ropes that were tied to the patient's pelvis and head. It used very strong traction. The bed also was equipped with a dialed scale to gauge how far weights had moved from the applied force. Maisonabe was unable to measure the resistance of the spinal column, and therefore found it very difficult to gauge the amount of weight required. His solution was to pull the patient's head manually to estimate the weights required for each patient and to err on the side of caution. One would increase tension by shortening the straps or ropes (Figure 14).

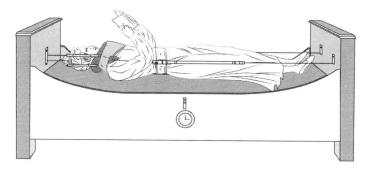

Figure 14. Extension bed by Maisonabe.

Many doctors were strongly against the use of extension beds, causing much controversy at the time. Some even accused proponents of "self-interest and poor physiological knowledge."[72]

Ambrose Paré, a famous French army surgeon, is considered the father of modern surgery and treatment with prostheses and supportive orthotic devices. He developed the first scoliosis brace in the 16th century. It was made of iron plates (Figure 15) . The brace was further developed in the 18th and 19th centuries in France and Germany (Figure 16).

---

72 Weiner, MF. "Abstract — Nature Publishing Group." 2009. 26 Apr. 2016. <http://www.nature.com/sc/journal/v47/n6/abs/sc200919a.html>

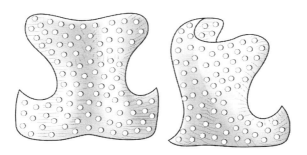

Figure 15. First support metal braces by Paré.

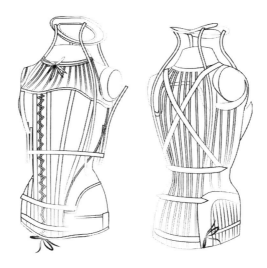

Figure 16. Hessing brace from Germany circa 1888.

In 1835, J. Hossard designed a corset that could be mechanically adjusted to correct spinal curvatures (Figure 17).

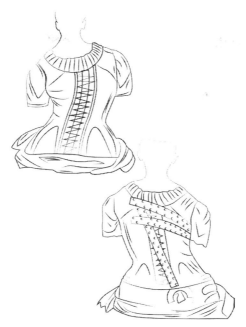

Figure 17. Corrective corset devices by Hossard.

Scoliosis Surgery

The first scoliosis surgery was attempted as early as 1839. Jules Guerin was the first to practice a transection (cutting across) of the paraspinal muscles to treat scoliosis. He believed scoliosis developed from an imbalance in the spinal muscles. The results were poor, which is why the method did not become widespread.[73]

L. Wullstein made an important contribution to the understanding of scoliosis in 1902 with his publication, *"Die Skoliose in ihrer Behandlung und Entstehung,"* which documented his clinical and experimental research on scoliosis (Figure 19).[74]

---

73 "Index of /paper_pdf — Osteopathic Research Web." 2012. 20 Apr. 2016 <http://www.osteopathic-research.com/paper_pdf/>

74 "Die Skoliose in Ihrer Behandlung und Entstehung nach ..." 2013. 20 Apr. 2016 <http://www.worldcat.org/title/skoliose-in-ihrer-behandlung-und-entstehung-nach-klinischen-und-experimentellen-studien/oclc/21218666>

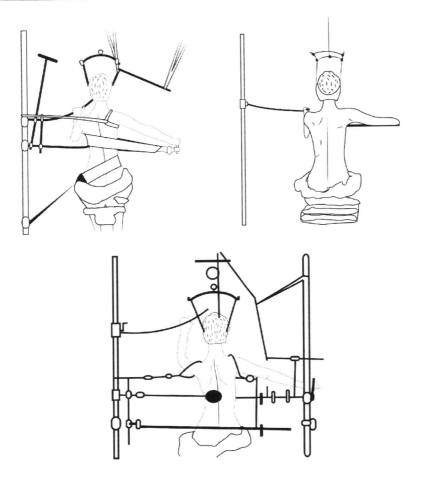

Figure 19. Wullstein scoliosis therapy.

Treatments in the 19th and early 20th centuries included exercises for strengthening the back muscles, as well as casts, braces and combinations of traction, suspension, bracing and postural corrections.

Here are illustrations of photographs from 1879-1883, taken by Augusta Zetterling, one of the first female photographers in Sweden.[75] Her subject was a girl with scoliosis. (Figure 22). She is shown wearing an early corrective brace in one of the photographs.

75 "Scoliosis | Wunderkammer." 2012. 20 Apr. 2016 <http://wunderkammer.ki.se/images/scoliosis>

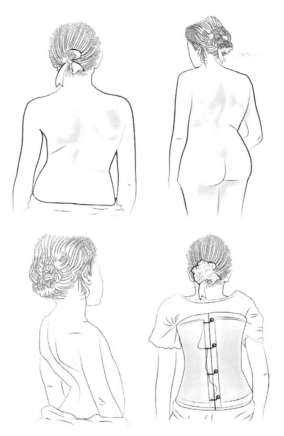

Figure 20. Illustration of photos taken by Augusta
Zetterling of a scoliosis patients.

Chapter 22. Scoliosis Bracing: Then and Now

I see many cases of children that have been subjected to years of wearing a scoliosis brace, and the curve has continued to progress. In this chapter, I will give you a background on scoliosis bracing and provide evidence as to why bracing can sometimes be a poor choice for adolescent idiopathic scoliosis. Other times, it can be the best option.

Conventional scoliosis braces are not designed to correct curves. While some reduction occasionally does take place, the primary goal is to slow progress and stabilize the existing curve size. If your surgeon has already determined that surgery will be necessary, he may place your child in an older-style brace simply to slow curve progression until the bones are developed enough to hold the hooks and screws that the surgery rods are attached to. He doesn't really care if the brace "works" because he has already determined that he will be operating on this child. Bad idea!

How about using a really effective custom-designed brace that has a solid chance of helping the child? Of course not every case will respond adequately to even the best of brace designs and a small percentage of the braced children will eventually require surgery, but brace technology has changed significantly in recent years. We have new materials, new approaches, new design methods, new manufacturing methods. The brace of even 10 years ago is radically deficient compared to the best of the braces available today. Unfortunately, almost all orthopedic surgeons and orthotists (Orthotists design and fabricate medical supportive devices and measure and fit patients for them) are still using and promoting outdated designs.

There are two groups of patients who can use scoliosis bracing. The first group includes young people who have not reached skeletal maturity. Their braces are meant to be used while the spine is still growing. The second group comprises skeletally mature patients of various ages and genders (most girls' skeletons mature earlier than boys).

Before we look at modern bracing approaches, let's look back in time to see how this concept of bracing has evolved.

History of Scoliosis Bracing

The history of the scoliosis back brace begins with Ambrose Paré, who is said to be the physician to first use an orthosis. His brace resembled a metal corset and was made by an armorer in 1575.[76] (Figure 1).

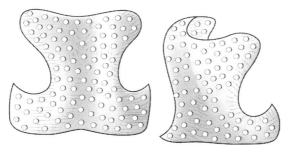

Figure 1. Metal braces by Paré.

Paré decided it was not useful once the person reached skeletal maturity. In 1945, Walter Blount introduced the **Milwaukee Brace** for post-operative immobilization of scoliosis patients. It was adapted later for non-surgical treatment, becoming one of the most commonly used – but not the most effective – scoliosis braces today.

Modern bracing has its foundation in the work of Dr. Jacques Chêneau of Toulouse, France. Chêneau constructed a derotation brace out of polyeth-

76 Fayssoux, RS. "A History of Bracing for Idiopathic Scoliosis in North America." 2010. 20 Apr. 2016.<http://www.ncbi.nlm.nih.gov/pubmed/19462214>

ylene that was presented in 1979 by Professor H. H. Matthiass of Münster as the **"Chêneau Brace"** (Chêneau-Toulouse-Münster, CTM) (Figure 2, C).

During the past few years, Dr. Rigo of Barcelona has furthered the development of the original Chêneau brace by combining his new classification of scoliosis to further customize brace design. His hybrid is called the **Rigo System Chêneau Brace** (RSC Brace) (Figure 2, B).

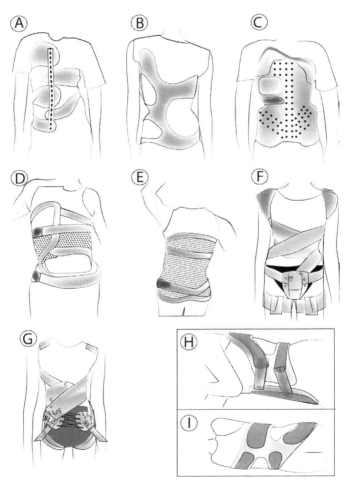

Figure 2. A: Chêneau Light Brace, B: Rigo-System Chêneau (RSC) Brace, C: Chêneau, D&E: Wilmington Brace, F&G: SpineCor Brace, H&I: Providence Brace.

Today, there are a variety of scoliosis braces many of which are named after the city of their original design. Some examples are the **Boston Brace**, the **Milwaukee Brace**, the **Lyon Brace,** and the **Wilmington Brace** (Figure 2, D and E). Other braces on the market include the **ART Brace**, the **SPoRT Brace** and the **ScoliBrace**. There are also "part-time" scoliosis braces, designed to be worn only at night, including the **Providence Brace** (Figure 2, H and I) and the **Charleston Brace**.

The **SpineCor Brace** (Figure 2, F and G), developed at Sainte-Justine Hospital by Spine Corp. in 1992, is considered a "dynamic corrective brace." Dynamic corrective braces use soft elastic materials and claim to do more than simply stabilize the progression of scoliosis.[77] The independent research on soft braces (such as SpineCor) reveal that this type of brace is compressive on the curve and therefore of questionable efficacy on larger curves (above 25 degrees Cobb). Because compressive bands are worn which pull the shoulders downward, they tend to increase the pressure on the curve. Furthermore, the argument that a soft brace overcomes the discomfort issues of a hard brace has proven to be unfounded.[78] Because the soft brace requires the use of a tight girdle to anchor the brace, it too has wearer discomfort issues.

A new type of brace has been released recently, and I use it in cases of rapidly progressing curves that are not responsive to an exercise-based approach, as well as in certain types of postural side shift and with adults who are experiencing pain as gravity takes its toll. I use the brace in approximately 30 percent of the cases that I treat.

This advanced and versatile brace can be used in infantile and adolescent cases – even with patients who are skeletally mature. Each design follows a corrective mirror-image principle applied to each patient's specific imbalance.

---

77 "SpineCor Dynamic Corrective Brace." 2013. 22 Apr. 2016 <http://www.spine-cor.com/ForProfessionals/SpineCorDynamicCorrectiveBrace.aspx>

78 Guo, J. "A Prospective Randomized Controlled Study on the Treatment ..." 2014. 26 Apr. 2016. <http://link.springer.com/article/10.1007%2Fs00586-013-3146-1>

"How Does Scientific Research Evaluate Bracing?"

There is much conflicting research on the efficacy of traditional scoliosis braces. Some studies have shown very little difference between patients who wore the scoliosis brace for the prescribed time and those who wore it rarely, if at all. Other studies have demonstrated patients who have been successfully stabilized for years by wearing a scoliosis brace constantly. And still there are other studies on patients who wore the scoliosis brace for 23 hours out of every day, seven days a week, and still continued to worsen.

A peer-reviewed study from 2007, published in the *SPINE* journal, compared 15 separate scoliosis brace studies **(evaluating the older styles of braces like the Boston and Milwaukee bracing systems)** with three observation-only studies and stated:

> *"Observation-only or scoliosis brace treatment showed no clear advantage of either approach. Furthermore one can not recommend one approach over another to prevent scoliosis surgery."*

They gave these outdated scoliosis brace treatments a "D" grade relative to observation because of *"troubling inconsistent or inconclusive studies on any level."*

In another article published by *SPINE* in 2001 stated, *"Since 1991, scoliosis bracing has not been recommended for children with adolescent idiopathic scoliosis."*

> *"If bracing does not reduce the proportion of children with AIS who require surgery for cosmetic improvement of their deformity, it cannot be said to provide a meaningful advantage to the patient or the community."*[79]

The *Journal of Pediatric Orthopedics* 2007 edition published a study focusing on the professional opinion of scoliosis brace efficacy in comparison to no treatment. The results show almost 50 percent of the respondents to the

---

[79] Goldberg, CJ. "Adolescent Idiopathic Scoliosis: the Effect of Brace Treatment ..." 2001. 26 Apr. 2016. <http://www.ncbi.nlm.nih.gov/pubmed/11148644>

study felt bracing had no effect on the scoliotic spine, and yet 100 percent still recommended scoliosis bracing as a treatment.

All the controversy over the effectiveness of bracing is somewhat misleading. Most negative information you read online is referring to the older brace systems and NOT the modern corrective designs. You never will find a doctor claiming that these older bracing systems consistently reduce or correct scoliosis; rather, the debate is over whether or not wearing that type of brace will prevent the scoliosis from getting worse. When doctors state that bracing "works," what they're really saying is that it stabilizes the scoliosis, keeping it at its current position. Most doctors will insist that bracing does "work" – with proper compliance. Recommended compliance is typically to wear the scoliosis back brace 20 hours per day, every day, for many years. If this seems a little extreme to you, you're not alone.

In a study published in the *American Journal of Orthopedics*, 60 percent of the patients surveyed felt that bracing had handicapped their life, and 14 percent felt it had left a psychological scar. Now you can understand why I use bracing only in the cases that I believe will not be responsive to my exercise-based program of care!

Many times I provide a trial period of exercise-based treatment only. If I see the patient would benefit from bracing, I will discuss this with the parents. A custom-designed exercise approach is FIRST. The best of the modern braces is the SECOND option. And, surgery should only be considered as a LAST resort!

For over 500 years the traditional scoliosis back brace has subsisted. Now three-dimensional imaging technology, combined with modern materials and mirror image design, has made bracing an effective approach – WHEN NEEDED. It is for these reasons, and based on the evidence, that we use bracing in a selected segment of our patients. Yes, there is a call for bracing at times, but it's much less common among patients using an exercise-based treatment program.

Chapter 23. The History of Scoliosis Surgery

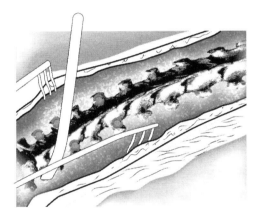

Scoliosis surgery is one of the most complicated orthopedic surgical procedures performed on children. It is also performed on adults, though not as frequently. When conservative treatments like scoliosis exercise programs or bracing are not effective in preventing the progression of the scoliosis, surgery may be prescribed to stop the curve's progression. Surgery may even be prescribed sooner if the curve progression rate is rapid during a short period of time.

Surgery recommendations for adolescents whose growth is complete vary from a low of 25-40 degrees all the way up to 60-70 degrees, depending on the specialist asked. The variation is due to differing philosophies of the orthopedic surgeons specializing in scoliosis. While some families will opt for surgery at the lower threshold to correct cosmetic issues, others will refrain from surgery unless the curve size develops to be very large (over 80 degrees) **AND** there begins to be evidence of heart and/or lung dysfunction.

History of Scoliosis Surgery

The first scoliosis surgeries were conducted by a French surgeon named Jules Rene Guerin in 1865.[80] This initial surgical attempt to help scoliosis patients involved severing the muscles and tendons of 1,349 patients. This resulted in horrific effects and lead to what many consider to be the first recorded instance of medical dispute and one of the most famous orthopedic lawsuits.

Dr. Russell Hibbs performed the first spinal fusion scoliosis surgery at the New York Orthopedic Hospital in 1914. The inventor of spinal fusion surgery; he had been performing the operation on other spinal deformities for three years before applying it to the treatment of scoliosis.[81] [82]

By 1941, spinal fusion operations for idiopathic scoliosis were common. The fusions were initially developed to treat tuberculosis which can affect the spinal bones. Most surgeons (60%) used supplemental bone grafts, often from the shin bones. An approximately 25 percent final curve correction was achieved. A high complication rate was associated with these early surgeries.

Twenty years later Paul Harrington introduced the first use of implanted steel rods to straighten scoliosis surgically. These hooks and rods are known as a spinal instrumentation system. Harrington's original concept was to use spinal instrumentation without fusion.[83]

---

80 "Jules Guérin – Wikipedia." 26 Apr. 2016 <https://sv.wikipedia.org/wiki/Jules_Gu%C3%A9rin>

81 "The History of Lumbar Spine Stabilization." 2005. 26 Apr. 2016 <http://www.burtonreport.com/infspine/SurgStabilSpineHistory.htm>

82 "Spinal Fusion: MedlinePlus Medical Encyclopedia." 2006. 26 Apr. 2016 <https://www.nlm.nih.gov/medlineplus/ency/article/002968.htm>

83 "Paul Randall Harrington — Wikipedia, the Free Encyclopedia." 2011. 26 Apr. 2016 <https://en.wikipedia.org/wiki/Paul_Randall_Harrington>

Due to poor results with just rods, ihs protocol changed to spinal fusion in conjunction with the Harrington rods. The Harrington Rod procedure was developed in the 1950s. A single inflexible steel rod secured the straightened spine, and bone was grafted from the patient's hip and placed into the vertebral spaces to stimulate a fusion. This surgery was performed through the back and lead to loss of all flexibility in the full length of the fusion. The surgery lasted between eight and 12 hours, and recovery was slow and difficult.

The patient would be confined to bed for three to six months in a full body cast from the neck to below the hips and another six months in a hard plastic jacket similar to today's **Wilmington Brace**.

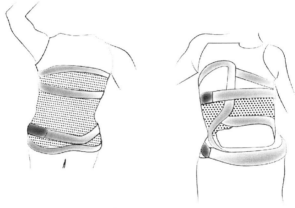

Wilmington Brace

By the mid-70s, the Harrington method often was performed using two rods to correct the upper and lower curves.

Cotrel and Dubousset developed the pedicle screw system known as Cotrel-Dubousset (CD) instrumentation. It was the first system that allowed for derotation of the vertebral bodies which corrected scoliosis in the sagittal (front to back) plane in addition to the coronal/lateral (side to side). Although correction rates achieved by posterior pedicle-screw are good overall, the rate of post-scoliosis surgery complications is very high.[84]

84 "Lumbar Fusion | University of Maryland Medical Center." 26 Apr. 2016 <http://umm.edu/programs/spine/health/guides/lumbar-fusion>

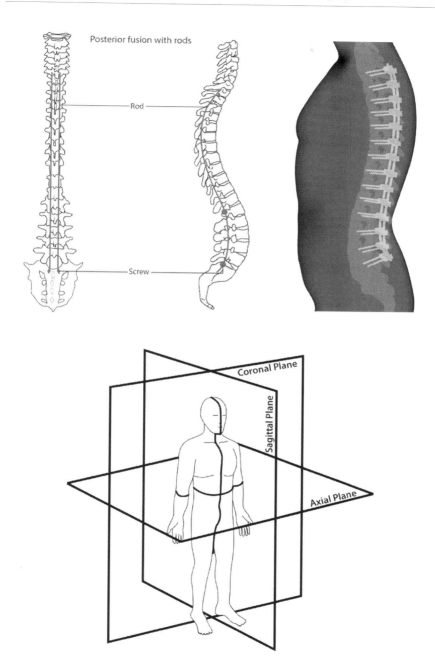

One study found that 68 percent of patients experienced minor or major severe complications. Another study determined that there is no significant improvement to surgical outcomes by using the C-D system over Harrington rods, while the newer C-D system is significantly more expensive.[85]

There is now a new innovation in scoliosis surgery that was developed at Shriners Hospital in Philadelphia. This new surgical approach is called Vertebral Body Tethering. There is no fusion and the spine retains mobility. Another benefit is the small incisions used in most cases. Not all scoliosis is able to benefit from this technique, and there are only a small number of surgeons employing the approach. As of early 2016, the procedure had not achieved FDA approval and is deemed experimental.

While there is obviously a place for surgery in the treatment of scoliosis, when curve sizes are small to moderate, or the family is opposed to surgery, exercise-based programs can be a viable alternative to bracing and/or surgery. Exercise-based programs include not only the CLEAR method, but also Méthode Lyonnaise, DoboMed, Functional Independent Treatment for Scoliosis (FITS), Side Shift exercises, Vojta method, Schroth (and its various offshoots), SEAS, McAviney, and CBP.

Since 2002, the CLEAR Institute has implemented innovative treatment methods that correct scoliosis without the use of bracing or surgery.[86] This worldwide group of 42 highly trained professionals have implemented a chiropractic and physiotherapeutic treatment system that combines in-office treatment with at-home exercises and rehabilitation designed to keep forward momentum of treatment when the patient is not in the office. While the CLEAR treatment model was designed to be used independently of bracing, it is used effectively in conjunction with scoliosis bracing by a segment of the CLEAR doctors. There are still a percentage of cases of scoliosis that have no alternative but surgery (i.e. curves of very large size that create respiratory stress or heart conditions). Research estimates this rare need as one-tenth of one percent (0.1%) of scoliosis patients.[87]

---

85 Modi, HN. "Scoliosis and Spinal Disorders | Pre-publication history ..." 2009. 26 Apr. 2016. <http://www.scoliosisjournal.com/content/4/1/11/prepub>

86 "CLEAR Scoliosis Institute." 2011. 26 Apr. 2016 <https://www.clear-institute.org/>

87 Labelle, H. "Screening for Adolescent Idiopathic Scoliosis: an ... — NCBI." 2013. 26 Apr. 2016. <http://www.ncbi.nlm.nih.gov/pmc/articles/PMC3835138/>

Chapter 24. Lung Function and Scoliosis

Because the thoracic spine is part of the thoracic cage which stores vital organs, such as the heart and lungs, significant scoliosis in the thoracic spine can affect heart and lung function. Studies have shown a significant correlation between lung and heart function and the degree of scoliosis in patients with very large thoracic-dominant scoliosis. Here we are talking about scoliosis greater than 80 degrees.

> *"Twenty-two (22%) of 98 patients complained of shortness of breath during everyday activities compared with eight (15%) of 53 controls. An increased risk of shortness of breath was also associated with the combination of a Cobb angle greater than 80 degrees and a thoracic apex (adjusted odds ratio, 9.75; 95% CI, 1.15-82.98). Sixty-six (61%) of 109 patients reported chronic back pain compared with 22 (35%) of 62 controls (P =.003). However, of those with pain, 48 (68%) of 71 patients and 12 (71%) of 17 controls reported only little or moderate back pain."[94]*

Another study which corroborates these findings concludes, "Pulmonary and cardiac function was significantly correlated with the degree of scoliosis in patients with thoracic-dominant scoliosis."[89]

---

88 Weinstein, SL. "Health and Function of Patients with Untreated ... - NCBI." 2003. 26 Apr. 2016. <http://www.ncbi.nlm.nih.gov/pubmed/12578488>

89 Huh, S. "Cardiopulmonary Function and Scoliosis Severity in ... — NCBI." 2015. 26 Apr. 2016. <http://www.ncbi.nlm.nih.gov/pmc/articles/PMC4510355/>

Does scoliosis surgery fix this type of lung problem? Unfortunately the answer is usually "No."

In *Scoliosis and the Human Spine*, Dr. Martha Hawes, Ph.D., the author, talks candidly about the impact of surgery on lung dysfunction:

> "If pulmonary dysfunction were a consequence of spinal curvature per se, then improving the magnitude of curvature would be predicted to result in a corresponding improvement in pulmonary function. However, instead [the pulmonary dysfunction] is due to a secondary loss of skeletal mobility. Further reductions in spinal and skeletal mobility beyond those associated with the spinal deformity being treated is one of the complications of spinal fusion surgery. Therefore it is not surprising that **surgically-induced improvement in Cobb Angle is not correlated with a matching increases in respiratory function and that pulmonary function may in fact decline after surgery** (Bjure, 1969; Goldberg, 2002; Katz and Kumar, 1983; Kinnear, 1992; Lenke, 1995; Lenke, 2002; Sakic, 1992; Upadhyay, 1994)."

> "In summary, after recovery from a significant decline in respiratory function due to the surgery per se there ultimately may be a slight improvement in pulmonary function, or there may be a decrease, or there may be no change at all (Kishan, 2007; Vedantam, 2000; Koumbourlis, 2006; McCool and Rochester, 2000; Newton and Wenger, 2001; Seaton, 2000). **Physicians are advised to let their patients know that improved pulmonary function, let alone a significant improvement, is not a reasonable expectation of spine surgery** (Bowen, 1995)."

> "Impact of spine surgery on signs & symptoms of spinal deformity," again by Hawes, states: "For most patients, there is little or no improvement in pulmonary function." Hawes also mentions that, "Since 1995, only 9 of 93 papers on "scoliosis surgery" have included spirometry to measure pulmonary function as part of the outcome. With one exception, these recent reports confirm previous studies indicating that, **irrespective of severity of curvature or surgical approach, improved curvature magnitude does not result in significantly improved *VC, **TLC, or exercise capacity.**"[90]

---

90 *Vital Capacity, **Total Lung Capacity

Let's connect the dots here... What does decreased lung function due to very large scoliosis mean with regard to lifespan? How does decreased lung function effect the lifespan of patients with very large curves?

Lets look at the Framingham Heart Study data which concluded that **"your lungs are the number one predictor of death."** This is not a scoliosis study, however the conclusions are very valuable for understanding the importance of proper lung function.

The Framingham Heart Study is a medical study that started in 1948 and has followed a population of thousands for six decades. The original researchers recruited over 5,200 men and women from Framingham, Mass. At that time, study participants were free of any cardiovascular disease.

In 1971, the study enrolled adult children of original participants and their spouses, and in 1994 additional subjects were enrolled in order to create a more diverse study population. In 2002, a third generation – the grandchildren of the original participants – started enrolling.

The Framingham Study is one of the oldest, largest and most prestigious ongoing medical studies in the world. One of the focuses of their study was the long-term predictive effects of vital capacity and forced exhalation volume (lung function) as a primary marker for lifespan.

Here's what the Framingham doctors wrote:

> *"Pulmonary function measurement (a measure of lung function) appears to be an indicator of general health and vigor and literally a measure of living capacity... Long before a person becomes terminally ill, vital capacity can predict lifespan. The Framingham examinations' predictive powers were as accurate over the 30-year period as were more recent exams."*[91]

In other words, lung capacity predicted lifespan as accurately as any other exams.

---

91 Mahmood, SS. "The Framingham Heart Study and the Epidemiology ... — NCBI." 2014. 25 Apr. 2016. <http://www.ncbi.nlm.nih.gov/pmc/articles/PMC4159698/>

Chapter 25. Surgery is Rarely Needed. It Should be a Choice!

Adolescent idiopathic scoliosis (AIS) affects 3-4 percent of children aged 10–16 years. Rather than grow upward, the spine curves outward, forming into a "C" or "S" shape. Ribs can also begin to protrude from the side of the body due to the curvature in the spine. During a routine examination, these signs of scoliosis will be spotted, and an x-ray will be taken to confirm that there is a curve in the spine.

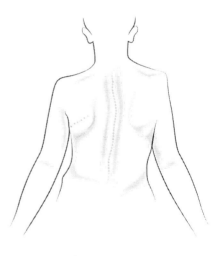

It is my opinion that all cases of scoliosis require early-stage treatment consisting of exercises specifically prescribed for the individual curve pattern. However, the currently practiced medical approach is that if your spinal curve is less than 25 degrees, check-ups are conducted by a doctor every four to six months to see whether the curve is getting worse, but no other treatment is provided or suggested! If the curve is between 25 and 40 degrees, the medical model is to institute treatment of bracing. When the curve becomes larger than 45-50 degrees, or if it is already greater than 50 degrees and likely to progress, surgery is then often prescribed **as if it were medically necessary!**

The research shows that unless scoliosis is above 50-60 degrees there is typically no detectable abnormalities of lung function. Unless the curve size exceeds 90 degrees, there will rarely be significant problems with the lungs or heart. In other words, this major surgery is done mostly for elective, cosmetic reasons. NOT for medical necessity![92] (Koumbourlis, 2006; Redding et al., 2011; Lonstein, 1994)

The lungs should be evaluated in all cases of significant scoliosis so that any issues with function are noted as early as possible. Computerized spirometry is the appropriate technology to use in thorough lung function assessment.

The most common methods of scoliosis surgery are highly invasive and require doctors to make a large incision down the back and spread open the ribs. One or more steel alloy or titanium rods are inserted – along with hooks, pins and pieces of bone to secure the remaining bones and fuse the spine into place in an attempt to prevent it from curving further. The surgical procedure is then followed by a painful recovery period that leaves patients with very large scars.

Very few hospitals across the country are now offering newer experimental techniques for scoliosis surgery, procedures such as tethering, stapling and anterior approaches through the chest rather than the back. It is purported that patients opting for these experimental surgical methods have less pain, need less narcotics, are less sedated, and have a quicker recovery with a shorter hospital stay. However, these surgeries cannot be performed on children with severe scoliosis. So, only patients with mild to moderate scoliosis are eligible for these new procedures. Sure this is an improvement to the older rod and fusing surgery, but these new surgical methods are still only offered at a few hospitals, and at the time of this writing have not been approved by the FDA.

Rather than making strides in scoliosis surgery, perhaps the focus should be on establishing a better medical model. The better approach would be one that doesn't wait until surgery is the only option, but instead takes a proactive exercise-based approach.

---

92 Tsiligiannis, Theofanis, and Theodoros Grivas. "Pulmonary Function in Children with Idiopathic Scoliosis." *Scoliosis* 7.1 (2012): 7. 22 Apr. 2016.

> *"One of the things that became clear, and which was actually rather disturbing, was the fact that there was a view which was being expressed by people whose scientific credentials you can't question."*
>
> **– Thabo Mbeki**
>
> (Discussing the medical profession's reaction to the AIDS epidemic in Africa.)

Chapter 26. A Disturbing Report on Scoliosis Surgery

Yes, there is a time when surgery is absolutely the right thing to do in scoliosis treatment. When severe adolescent idiopathic scoliosis progresses to a point at which lung and heart function are compromised, surgery can become a necessary intervention. Spinal fusion surgery on a large scoliosis is a very complex and invasive medically nec-

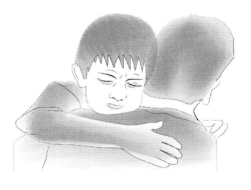

essary surgical procedure that can result in strong postoperative pain. A 2013 study detailed the experiences of patients (ages 8-25) who underwent corrective spinal surgery between 2004-2007, and the results were an unsettlingly consistent tale of extreme pain, debilitating nausea and an overwhelming sense of helplessness.[93]

---

93 Rullander, AC. "Young People's Experiences with Scoliosis Surgery: a Survey ..." 2013. 26 Apr. 2016. <http://www.ncbi.nlm.nih.gov/pubmed/24247313>

The study found, on average, most postoperative pain was described as severe and lasting for roughly five days. Of those adolescents, 60 percent also reported "persistent pain or recent onset pain 5-12 months after surgery." Patients from the study detailed experiences of mismanagement and unbearable pain while getting in and out of bed, standing and during chest tube removal.

"I felt like I was hung up on meat hooks."
"Sometimes it feels like a knife is cutting into my back."

As one can imagine, pain management is an essential part of recovery and can involve epidural, intravenous and also spinal analgesics. However, these medications come with their own sets of side effects: nausea, constipation, pruritus (itching), urinary retention, sedation, respiratory depression and decreased blood pressure. Nausea was another common complaint. The nausea persisted for an average of three days, though some patients experienced it for the duration of their hospital stay or even after they left. Parents reported drug treatment as ineffective and that the nausea only subsided when opioid medication doses were decreased. Some patients reported not eating while in the hospital because of nausea, and some even felt the nausea was worse than the pain.

The most heartbreaking detail of this study were the parents' feelings of helplessness as their children were suffering. Parents and patients described inadequacies of nursing staff, failure of pain control equipment, anxiety, nightmares and too much time spent waiting for assistance. The authors indicate that "symptoms of post traumatic stress were vividly described in narrative interviews with some of the adolescents."

> *"She had fear in her eyes. We have never seen that expression before. She cannot express herself you know! I can't remember whether she screamed or moaned or if she stared at us with pure fear trying to say – help me!"*

> *"Everything was OK until the catheter with analgesics stopped functioning. After that there were several difficult days with severe pain. My daughter has had nightmares about pain since then."*

"It was terrible to see my daughter having so much pain and not being able to help her."[94]

What's shocking though is that parents and patients alike rated their overall hospital stay as satisfactory. Researchers suggested such a discrepancy may exist because satisfaction was based on other factors, including that they expected such an experience.

Since this study, pain management techniques have been modified to include "patient-controlled epidural analgesia." However, the authors are quick to add that the most painful instances were when the epidural catheters failed and when patients were switched from the catheters to oral medications.

From Physician-Patient Alliance for Health & Safety (PPAHS.ORG):

"Patient Controlled Analgesia (PCA) pumps were developed to address the problem of under medication. They are used to permit the patient to self-administer small doses of narcotics (usually Morphine, Dilaudid, Demerol, or Fentanyl) into the blood or spinal fluid at frequent intervals. PCA pumps are commonly used after surgery to provide a more effective method of pain control than periodic injections of narcotics."[101]

Another 2013 study on postoperative pain from spinal fusion surgery assessed pain scores, use of opioids, and the recovery process. It stated:

"The standard of care for pain management for spine surgery in children consists of continuous infusion of intravenous (IV) morphine supplemented with patient-controlled analgesia (PCA). However, to achieve satisfactory pain control with this method, high doses of opioids must be administered. Unfortunately, use of opioids is associated with

94 Rullander, Anna-Clara et al. "Young People's Experiences with Scoliosis Surgery: a Survey of Pain, Nausea, and Global Satisfaction." *Orthopaedic Nursing* 32.6 (2013): 327-333. Print.

95 "Patient Controlled Analgesia (PCA) Pumps: The Basics." 2015. 25 Apr. 2016 <http://www.ppahs.org/2012/05/patient-controlled-analgesia-pca-pumps-the-basics/>

serious adverse effects, including nausea, vomiting, pruritus, sedation, and respiratory depression, which often delay patient recovery."[96]

Surgery for all but the largest curve (0.1 percent of scoliosis cases) should be called what it really is: "elective spinal fusion surgery." ELECTIVE, not NECESSARY. Parents need to be fully informed that surgery is a treatment choice and is rarely a necessity. You do have a choice to provide a surgical solution to your child, or not! A custom-designed exercise program and over-corrective bracing when appropriate are just as valid a choice in the vast majority of scoliosis cases in children.

Let's look at two excerpts from two different *Spine* articles about the discouraging outcome of some spinal implant removals:

"Despite bony fusion, loss of correction between 10 degrees and 26 degrees was observed in three patients after instrumentation removal."[97]

"Spinal implant removal after long posterior fusion in adults may lead to spinal collapse and further surgery. Removal of instrumentation should be avoided or should involve partial removal of the prominent implant."[98]

That's hard to read, isn't it?

---

96 Reynolds, RA. "Postoperative Pain Management after Spinal Fusion Surgery ..." 2013. 26 Apr. 2016. <http://www.ncbi.nlm.nih.gov/pubmed/24436846>

97 Hahn, Frederik, Reinhard Zbinden, and Kan Min. "Late Implant Infections Caused by Propionibacterium Acnes in Scoliosis Surgery." *European Spine Journal* 14.8 (2005): 783-788. Print.

98 Deckey, Jeffrey E, and David S Bradford. "Loss of Sagittal Plane Correction after Removal of Spinal Implants." *Spine* 25.19 (2000): 2453-2460. Print.

> *"We live in a world of constant juxtaposition between joy that's possible and pain that's all too common. We hope for love and success and abundance, but we never quite forget that there is always lurking the possibility of disaster."*
>
> **– Marianne Williamson**

Chapter 27. Can Spinal Rods, Hooks and Screws Break?

Steel alloy and even titanium rods can bend, break loose from their wires, or worse, break completely in two, necessitating further surgical intervention and removal of the rods.[99] Once the rod is removed, corrosion is found on two out of every three.[100]

Recent studies are showing concern about the possible toxic effect on the body of having a large metallic implant for decades. One study suggests that the presence of metallic particles from titanium-alloy pedicle screw hardware may be the cause of late-onset inflammatory response and late operative-site pain.[101]

99 "Scoliosis Surgery: Things to Consider-OrthoInfo — AAOS." 2011. 25 Apr. 2016 <http://orthoinfo.aaos.org/topic.cfm?topic=A00641>

100 Akazawa, Tsutomu et al. "Corrosion of Spinal Implants Retrieved from Patients with Scoliosis." *Journal of Orthopaedic Science* 10.2 (2005): 200-205. Print.

101 Kim, HD. "Electron Microprobe Analysis and Tissue Reaction ... — NCBI." 2007. 26 Apr. 2016. <http://www.ncbi.nlm.nih.gov/pmc/articles/PMC2857498/>

Though, complication due to metal hypersensitivity is rare, some studies suggest that cases involving implant-related metal sensitivity are underreported because they are difficult to diagnosis.[102] [103] [104] [105]

Prospective studies have shown a higher incidence of metal hypersensitivity in patients with implant failure.[106] Researchers suggest that metal hypersensitivity after spinal fusion should be suspected in patients with postoperative back pain and that an elaborate case history would lead to a correct diagnosis.[107]

> *"The brief answer to our initial question is yes, patients can be allergic to hardware if they have a pre-existing allergy to the materials that make up the hardware (titanium, stainless steel, etc.). Your surgical team will do a thorough investigation of your existing allergies prior to your procedure to avoid any potential allergic reactions after surgery. However, certain allergies can develop over time. So a person who has already had spinal hardware put in place can potentially develop an allergy to it years down the line.*
>
> *An allergic reaction can crop up in the form of headaches, pain in the back and extremities, fever, and other symptoms. If you notice*

102 Thyssen, Jacob Pontoppidan et al. "The Association Between Metal Allergy, Total Hip Arthroplasty, and Revision: A Case-Control Study." *Acta Orthopaedica* 80.6 (2009): 646-652. Print.

103 Shang, X. "Metal Hypersensitivity in Patient with Posterior Lumbar Spine ..." 2014. 25 Apr. 2016. <http://bmcmusculoskeletdisord.biomedcentral.com/articles/10.1186/1471-2474-15-314>

104 Jokar, M. "Epidemiology of Vasculitides in Khorasan Province, Iran." 2015. 26 Apr. 2016. <http://www.ncbi.nlm.nih.gov/pmc/articles/PMC4487463/>

105 Thyssen, Jacob Pontoppidan et al. "The Association Between Metal Allergy, Total Hip Arthroplasty, and Revision: A Case-Control Study." *Acta Orthopaedica* 80.6 (2009): 646-652. Print.

106 Frigerio, E. "Metal Sensitivity in Patients with Orthopaedic Implants: a ..." 2011. 26 Apr. 2016. <http://www.ncbi.nlm.nih.gov/pubmed/21480913>

107 Shang, Xianping et al. "Metal Hypersensitivity in Patient with Posterior Lumbar Spine Fusion: a Case Report and its Literature Review." *BMC Musculoskeletal Disorders* 15.1 (2014): 314. Print.

any severe symptoms after your spine surgery, be sure to contact your surgeon. It may be necessary to remove the spinal hardware to avoid any further complications.[108]

Below, is an illustration of two radiographs of an individual with broken spinal rods.

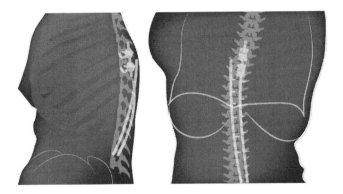

These x-rays show steel alloy rods that bent and broke while still inside the patient's body. Many surgeons will refuse to operate on this condition, leaving the patient with few options to alleviate their pain and suffering.[109]

Rod removal is usually considered when there is local pain over the site of a broken rod or from a prominent hook. Often, however, only part of a rod or one or more prominent hooks can be removed to relieve symptoms. The spinal fusions are often extremely solid and the new bone formation encases the rods and the hooks; therefore, removal of the entire rod may not be possible and one or more hooks may be left behind. The wound then needs two to three weeks to heal unless there is additional bone grafting needed.

Some curvatures continue to progress after spinal fusion due to broken rods or other instrument failure. In a paper about the role of Harrington instrumentation and posterior spine fusion in AIS patients, researcher T.S. Ren-

108 "Can You Be Allergic to Spine Hardware? | Dr. Stefano ..." 2014. 25 Apr. 2016 <http://sinicropispine.com/can-allergic-spine-hardware/>

109 "Scoliosis Surgery: Things to Consider-OrthoInfo — AAOS." 2011. 25 Apr. 2016 <http://orthoinfo.aaos.org/topic.cfm?topic=A00641>

shaw said that, *"One would expect that if the patient lives long enough, rod breakage will be a virtual certainty."110*

Furthermore, discomfort may occur when any pressure is placed against the back; this is especially problematical with newer bulky instrumentation implanted in thin patients, noted researcher H.R. Weiss in his 2008 study about AIS and surgery.111

Even with a solid fusion, a small percentage of Harrington rods subsequently fracture, due to micro-movement in daily activities. When rods break within two years of operation, it usually indicates fusion failure (pseudarthrosis) and it will need to be surgically repaired by more bone grafting and possible modification of the rods.112

Here are what those on online forums say when discussing complications, pain and discomfort from malfunctioning Harrington rods:

> *"My dad has had metal rods in his back since 1995. They are horrible. He is in so much more pain than before and now every doctor says there is nothing they can do for him b/c the rods can never come out. I am trying to get him into the mayo clinic but so far haven't had any luck. He lives in constant pain."*

To read more, go to: Orthopedics Forum – Broken Harrington Rod http://ehealthforum.com/health/topic10952.html#ixzz1x8lgiY42

> *"Hello, I too had scoliosis surgery when I was like 12 or 13. I am now 31. I had/have been having a lot of back pain. Last summer I went back to the dr. that did the surgery. That is when I found out that my rod is broken. I don't know when it happened. I just know I have con-*

---

110 Renshaw, T. S. "The Role of Harrington Instrumentation and Posterior Spine Fusion in the Management of Adolescent Idiopathic Scoliosis." *The Orthopedic Clinics of North America* 19.2 (1988): 257-267. Print.

111 Weiss, HR. "Adolescent Idiopathic Scoliosis – to Operate or Not? A ... — NCBI." 2008. 26 Apr. 2016. <http://www.ncbi.nlm.nih.gov/pmc/articles/PMC2572584/>

112 "Scoliosis Research Society." 2015. 25 Apr. 2016 <https://www.srs.org/chinese_sim/patient_and_family/the_aging_spine/pseudarthrosis.htm>

stant pain in my shoulder blade on up. So, unfortunately, yes the rod can break. But, I do not know the solution."

To read more, go to: National Scoliosis Foundation Forums http://www.scoliosis.org/forum/archive/index.php/t-210.html

"My daughter had her titanium Harrington rods removed on May 24th. She was two years post injury, and had constant, deep pain in her lower back. She was also constantly nauseated, making it difficult to eat."

To read more, go to: CareCure Forums – Removal of Harrington Rods at http://sci.rutgers.edu/forum/archive/index.php

"I was told the best they could do as a last resort would be to cut off pieces at each end of the break. To keep the broken halves from banging into each other. The rods were grafted/fused to my back using pieces of my hip. I was told to remove them would be extremely difficult and there was a good chance I'd be worse off afterward."

To read more, go to: Spina Bifida Connection Support Forum-Broken Harrington Rod Pics

http://spinabifidaconnection.com/archive/index.php/t-767.html

> *"We are built to conquer environment, solve problems, achieve goals, and we find no real satisfaction or happiness in life without obstacles to conquer and goals to achieve."*
>
> **– Maxwell Maltz**

Chapter 28. Can Patients View Scoliosis Surgery as 'Failed'?

If scoliosis surgery is so problematic, why is it that the majority of patients and their parents say they are pleased with the process?

A 2008 systematic review of the PubMed literature (Weiss et al.) discussed the possible influence of a psychological effect called "cognitive dissonance" in scoliosis surgery outcomes. Cognitive dissonance theory tells us that people have an internal psychological need to hold all their attitudes and beliefs in harmony and will not tolerate disharmony, or dissonance. Any psychological "discomfort" that comes from feeling like one has made a bad decision leads to an alteration of their attitudes, beliefs or behaviors to reduce the discomfort/anxiety and restore comfort/harmony.[113]

The authors of the study postulated that this type of discomfort may be occurring in patients who have a high rate of complications with scoliosis surgery, but still report they are happy with their decision. It also suggests that the rate of complications may be higher than reported.

> *"Instead of achieving long-term evidence for surgical treatment on a higher level and addressing the problems after surgery to attempt to improve patient's safety, the surgical community is presenting large numbers of papers describing HRQL (Health Related Quality of Life*

---

113 Weiss, Hans-Rudolf, and Deborah Goodall. "Rate of Complications in Scoliosis Surgery–a Systematic Review of the Pub Med Literature." *Scoliosis* 3.1 (2008): 1. 22 Apr. 2016.

Questionnaires) after surgery and related research. The problem with such studies however, is that they lack validity as they do not investigate the actual signs of scoliosis or the symptoms of the patient post surgery."

The studies containing psychological questionnaires may be compromised by the dissonance effect. Unable to face an inconsistency, such as being dissatisfied with a surgical procedure, a person will often change their attitude or action. Surgery is impossible to reverse, but subjective beliefs and public attitude can be altered more easily. In terms of research, this is important because a patient not satisfied with scoliosis surgery may not admit it."[114]

The authors of the study also give examples of the dissonance effect as reflected in scoliosis literature: *"Radiographic and physical measures of deformity do not correlate well with patients' and parents' perceptions of appearance. Patients and parents do not strongly agree on the cosmetic outcome of AIS surgery."* (Figure 1)

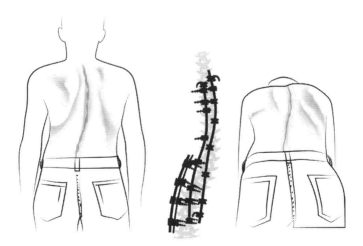

Figure 1. Patient's surgical outcome used as example in the study.

114 Weiss, HR, and HR Weiss. "Rate of Complications in Scoliosis Surgery – a ... — NCBI." 2008. 26 Apr. 2016. <http://www.ncbi.nlm.nih.gov/pmc/articles/PMC2525632/>

*"**Not the best clinical result with patient satisfaction**. This patient was satisfied although two operations have been necessary and the rib-hump and decompensation are still visible. **This satisfaction may be the result of the dissonance effect.**"*[115]

*"Today, from the patient's perspective, **health care professionals have more open questions than answers when approaching the subject of spinal surgery in patients with scoliosis**. For example; What are the long-term effects in the elderly; how long does the cosmetic effect of an operation last; is there a prospective controlled study clearly showing that scoliosis surgery really prevents progression in the long term; does the untreated patient really feel more impaired when progressing 10 degrees more in 20 years?"*[116]

Another more recent study by the same authors (Weiss et al., 2013) yet again addressed the lack of regard for cognitive dissonance in scoliosis literature. They suggest that spinal fusion for adolescent idiopathic scoliosis should only be considered when it is the rare curve that has progressed to a very severe degree or in patients with substantial psychological trauma due to scoliosis deformity. "However, this is rarely the case in a population treated conservatively according to the latest standards," Weiss said.

Most importantly, medical policy stresses the need for informed consent to document patient awareness and a surgeon's liability in patients requiring surgery. Patients need to be aware of the high percentage of long-term complications of fusion surgery and the extent of long-term complications.[117]

115 Weiss, HR, and Goodall, D. "Rate of Complications in Scoliosis Surgery – A ... — NCBI." 2008. 26 Apr. 2016. <http://www.ncbi.nlm.nih.gov/pmc/articles/PMC2525632/>

116 Weiss, HR. "Rate of Complications in Scoliosis Surgery – A Systematic ..." 2008. 26 Apr. 2016. <http://www.ncbi.nlm.nih.gov/pmc/articles/PMC2525632/>

117 "Risks and Long-Term Complications of Adolescent Idiopathic ..." 2013. 26 Apr. 2016 <http://www.oapublishinglondon.com/article/498>

"The stress the patient experiences due to the deformity must be documented," said Weiss. He also noted:

> "It is highly recommended that patients complete the preoperative patient awareness documentation regarding possible complications, sometimes presenting more than 20 years post-operatively. This documentation, in conjunction with the deformity-related stress level questionnaire, should be read carefully for full disclosure of long-term effects."[118]

The authors conclude, "A medical indication for AIS spinal fusion surgery does not exist, except in extreme cases. The rate of complications of spinal fusion surgery appears to increase with time. The risk/reward relationship of spinal fusion surgery is unfavourable for the AIS patient, except in rare cases. There is no evidence that spinal fusion surgery improves quality of life for AIS patients versus natural history. The risks and long-term costs, in terms of pain and suffering, after spinal fusion surgery exceeds what is reasonable for AIS patients, putting the common practice of surgery in question, except in extreme cases."[125]

---

118 "Risks and Long-Term Complications of Adolescent Idiopathic ..." 2013. 26 Apr. 2016 <http://www.oapublishinglondon.com/article/498>

119 "Risks and Long-Term Complications of Adolescent Idiopathic ..." 2013. 26 Apr. 2016 <http://www.oapublishinglondon.com/article/498>

Chapter 29. Orthopedists and the Potential for Conflict of Interest

Why Do Orthopedists Discourage Alternative Scoliosis Treatments Even When Patients Show Improvement from Them?

The medical approach to scoliosis treatment is to watch and wait, brace and then operate. During the "wait and see" period orthopedists generally do not advise patients of alternative treatment options and some even laugh or scoff at the suggestion. Patients are made to feel absurd if they want to pursue proactive or preventative treatments during this pre-brace/pre-surgery period and instead are advised to just sit idly while their curves progress until bracing or surgery become "necessary."

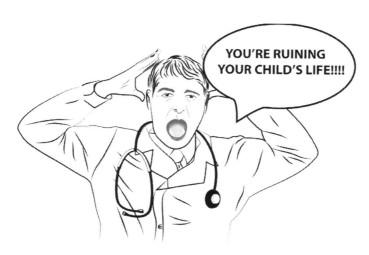

Some parents choose to research treatment and try alternative treatments anyway, but upon re-evaluation by their doctor they are told they are wasting their time! Parents are belittled, made to feel negligent, and even are harassed by their orthopedist. I have had patients tell me that their orthopedic surgeon screamed at them and told them they were ruining their child's life by seeking out an exercise-based program!

If there are fewer risks with alternative treatments, if these approaches are received while patients are in the "watch and wait" period, and if these treatments show improvement to the patient's scoliosis, then why is the medical community so against them?

DO ORTHOPEDISTS FAIL TO SUGGEST EARLY-INTERVENTION EXERCISE PROGRAMS OR OTHER ALTERNATIVE SCOLIOSIS TREATMENTS BECAUSE OF A CONFLICT OF INTEREST?

If you have surgery and it fails, exercise-based care programs will only be able to target the non-operated areas of the spine. Hooks, screws and stabilizing devices in your spine will impede exercise-based programs targeting those areas. If you have an exercise-based program that in the rare case is not successful, the surgeon will always be waiting for you. And… the improved mobility you gain from the specialized exercises and stretches would probably actually help the surgeon achieve a higher degree of correction.

In Martha C. Hawes' book *Scoliosis and the Human Spine* (2010), the University of Arizona professor and research scientist outlines what appears to be a conflict of interest in the medical community. The conflict centers upon the general lack of regard for exercise-based programs of scoliosis care and correction. Let's take a closer look.

DO NOTHING (Watch and Wait)

There has been a tremendous movement in the United States to screen for scoliosis. Why? So that it may be detected early in an attempt to intervene and treat before it progresses? If early intervention is the goal, why are we waiting?

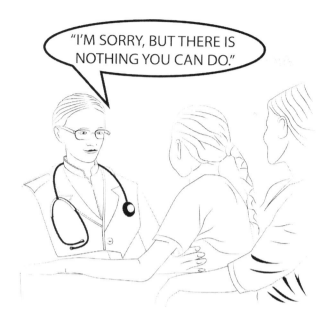

Dr. Hawes, Ph.D., who has scoliosis herself, said:

> "We have the wherewithal to diagnose spinal deformity at a Cobb magnitude of ten degrees or less, before it progresses to a serious problem that may cause pain, deformity, psychological dysfunction, and pulmonary problems throughout the patient's lifetime. But instead of making an effort to diagnose the underlying condition and take steps to stabilize or reverse the curvature at this relatively benign state (and despite longstanding basic and clinical research consistent with the hypothesis that this is entirely feasible), patients and parents formally are told to do NOTHING: Just keep coming in to an orthopedic surgeon's office every few months for another x-ray, and wait to see if it gets worse."[120]

---

120 Hawes, M.C. (2010). *Scoliosis and the Human Spine*. Tucson, Arizona: West Press. Print.

DON'T TRY ANYTHING ELSE

Not only are patients advised to do nothing, but they are discouraged from seeking alternative treatments or just informed that there is nothing that they can do.

> *"If individuals insist on searching out help on their own they are treated to condescension and insinuations that they are being irresponsible by trying 'scientifically unproven' treatments and refusing to accept the advice of professionals who know best (e.g. Keim, 1987; Lonstein, 1995a)." (Hawes 2010)*

If scoliosis screening is not geared to finding the curvature in its early stages and treating it before it progresses, then what is the intent? To merely refer more patients to orthopedic surgeons?

SCREENING LEADS to SURGERY

Since screening has begun, there have been more scoliosis surgeries performed. Is there a correlation?

If the goal were to decrease the number of adolescents subjected to spinal fusion surgery, then why are so many patients being referred to orthopedic surgeons? Since screening has been mandated, the average curve for which surgery is carried out decreased from a Cobb angle of 60 degrees to a Cobb angle of 42 degrees (Lonstein et al., 1987). This was done as a means to operate sooner rather than later under the assumption that moderate curves will inevitably become severe curves but, as Dr. Hawes points out in her book, "there are a lot more moderate (42° curves) than severe (> 60° curves) curvatures in the population." If one were to take a more cynical perspective, one could say that decreasing the average curve size indicated for surgery provides the surgeons with more cases on which to operate.

SURGEONS WOULD BE PUT OUT OF BUSINESS

In the United States in 2009, spinal surgery to correct adolescent idiopathic scoliosis ranked second only to appendicitis among children 10 to 17 years of age.[121]

> *"...if proactive therapies were found to be effective, orthopedic surgeons would be put out of business of spinal fusion surgery because there would be no progression to levels where such intervention might be warranted. (Hawes 2010)*

According to Martin et al., 2014 *Spine*, as cited online in a Health Advances article "Economic Impact of Novel Sublaminar Bands for AIS Fusion on Hospital Costs":

> *"U.S. hospital expenditures associated with AIS management surpassed $500 million in 2007 and have continued to increase dramatically in recent years. A recent analysis of adjusted U.S. hospital charges and costs associated with AIS spinal fusion surgery demonstrated that adjusted hospital charges and costs nearly doubled from 2001 to 2011, a significantly greater increase compared to other inpatient pediatric admissions, and likely indicative of a genuine change in hospital economics associated with AIS spinal fusions over that timeframe."[122]*

Why isn't there more research on alternative treatments to scoliosis? Why don't insurance companies cover these treatments?

---

121 Weinstein, SL. "Effects of Bracing in Adolescents with Idiopathic ... — NCBI." 2013. 20 Apr. 2016. <http://www.ncbi.nlm.nih.gov/pmc/articles/PMC3913566/>

122 Cole, D., Ilharreborde, B., Woo, R. (2015) *Retrospective Cost Effectiveness Analysis of Implanet Jazz Sublaminar Bands for Surgical Treatment of Adolescent Idiopathic Scoliosis.* 23 Apr. 2016. <http://www.implanet.com/wp-content/themes/theme-implanet/pdf/Health_Advances_Jazz_Cost-Effectiveness.pdf>

ORTHOPEDISTS HAVE TO DO SURGERY

There are many upsides to performing spinal fusion surgery as opposed to other forms of surgery, especially since scoliosis surgery is elective for many and arguably only done for "cosmetic" reasons.

"Orthopedists as a group relate the degree of satisfaction in their practice to the amount of surgery they get to do, and elective reconstructive surgery like spinal fusion is at the top of the list: High-skill, high-tech, very costly, covered by insurance, and no need to get up in the middle of the night to set messy fractures after car wrecks and suicide attempts." (Clawson 2001, Heckman 2001)

SOME ORTHOPEDISTS ARE PAID TO DEVELOP TECHNIQUES AND DEVICES FOR SCOLIOSIS SURGERY

There is also the added bonus of money and grants received by surgeons from the companies that supply the instrumentation that they use during spinal surgery.

"Some scoliosis surgeons receive royalties and research grants from the biomedical companies who make the ever-evolving array of spinal implantation devices." (Shufflebarger, 2001)

What is even more alarming is the rate at which these surgeries fail and require further medical intervention in the form of secondary surgical procedures, known amongst orthopedists as "salvage surgeries." This surgery can hardly be called "elective" as patients experiencing extreme pain and impairment are often left with no alternative but to undergo further procedures.

"What is more, the worst that can happen is that the surgery will fail (as it does, often), and additional costly, elective reconstructive surgery covered by insurance (or the personal savings of desperate parents) will be required. Such 'salvage' surgeries cost $100,000 or more."[123] (Hawes 2010)

---

123 Hawes, M.C. (2010). *Scoliosis and the Human Spine*. Tucson, Arizona: West Press. Print.

TOO MANY SURGEONS

Another major concern in the field of spinal fusion surgery is the large increase of orthopedic surgeons operating within the United States.

> "The ratio of orthopedist to U.S. population has increased, predictably, from 1 surgeon per 110,000 people in 1941 to 1:25,000 in 1980 to 1:15,150 in 1999 (Clawson 2001). Surveys have shown that when the ratio increases to 1:15,000 or more, there is a significant increase in the number of operations being performed per 100,000 people, with concern that more elective surgery is being done than necessary." (Hawes 2010)

Remember, almost all scoliosis surgery is truly elective, not done out of necessity. Hearing of pressure to have surgery because there is "not enough elective surgery to go around" is very disturbing. Shockingly, Hawes writes that spinal fusion surgery for teens with scoliosis was advertised on the radio in California in 2001!

> "An appearance of conflict of interest does not necessarily mean a conflict exists, and the vast majority of scoliosis surgeons undoubtedly are conscientious souls with a compassionate interest in their patients' welfare which overrides issues of personal gain. Indeed, leaders in the discipline have taken a strong stand in favor of the urgent need to establish and enforce clear ethical guidelines." (Shufflebarger 2001)

This is not to say that orthopedists or orthopedic surgeons are to be vilified for their practices, seeing as their advised treatment protocols are backed up by both peer-reviewed medical research and the insurance industry (that happen to fund said protocols). As Dr. Hawes also points out, one of the greatest contributors to scoliosis research, the Scoliosis Research Society (SRS), is comprised of several hundred orthopedic surgeons. Not only do they conduct research to better understand and treat scoliosis, but they also report issues within the field of surgical intervention for scoliosis.

DO SOMETHING!

So if patients are instructed to "wait and see," what alternative is there?

Do research!

Research other treatment options, read the scientific articles, check the blogs and forums, read the testimonials, talk with the patients. Do the work that the medical community won't do for you. Become an "expert" on your own condition, so you are prepared to discuss the issues.

Take a proactive approach to your health care! Don't be intimidated by your orthopedist. There may be a conflict of interest motivating their disapproval of alternative, exercise-based scoliosis care programs.

> "If we could give every individual the right amount of nourishment and exercise, not too little and not too much, we would have found the safest way to health."
>
> **– Hippocrates**

Chapter 30. The Best Exercises for Scoliosis

A custom designed scoliosis specific program of exercises can be a very effective part of a more comprehensive treatment plan for scoliosis. It's the type of exercise that is key! Exercise can be divided into two groups: isometric and isotonic.

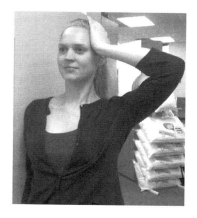

Isometrics are a way to exercise the muscles while in a stationary position. **Isometric exercise** is experienced by pushing or pulling a fixed object like a bar anchored to the wall or floor or even another body part that is stationary.

Research has shown that a muscle contraction during isometric exercise produces more force than a contraction generated by lifting weights. Isometric exercises can provide impressive results with minimal strain on the spine.

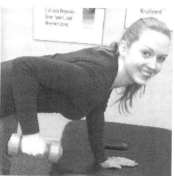

Isotonic exercise can be performed with free weights or with fixed equipment. Isotonic literally means equal tension. Isotonic contraction is when the tension remains constant as the muscle shortens or lengthens with body movement.

If you are unsure of the correct way to perform an exercise, please let your scoliosis specialist know immediately, as any exercise not done correctly will not have a positive impact on your spine. The type of exercise, body positioning, repetitions, and the order of the exercises must be individually designed for each patient. If you are going to put the time and effort into an exercise program to treat your scoliotic spine, be sure it is set up and followed correctly.

It is important to note that any scoliosis treatment program should include exercise as only one part of the whole program of care. Exercise and stretches alone will not achieve effective results. This is because scoliosis is linked to a problem in the automatic postural control centers of the brain. Research has revealed that in scoliotic spines, the brain doesn't "recognize" the scoliosis spine as out of alignment. Therefore, it doesn't trigger the spinal auto-correction mechanisms that would fix the scoliosis. Exercises will increase flexibility and strength, which may minimize pain and discomfort and improve posture visibly, but the curve size will stubbornly remain the same.[124]

Exercise treatments and stretches for scoliosis need to be performed in conjunction with a specific focus on creating a stimulus that triggers the brain to recognize that there is an abnormality and to auto-correct the spinal posture. This stimulus must affect the body at a subconscious level to create any meaningful changes in posture. If posture changes are accomplished willfully and consciously, as soon as patients take their attention off their posture, they will revert to the baseline posture which is supporting the scoliosis. In other words, any type of voluntary movement is overriding the subconscious automatic postural control centers in the brain and not allowing them to "learn" how to auto-correct the scoliosis spine.

---

124 Schimmel, JJP. "Adolescent Idiopathic Scoliosis and Spinal Fusion Do Not Substantially ..." 2015. 26 Apr. 2016. <http://www.ncbi.nlm.nih.gov/pmc/articles/PMC4459442/>

The most effective scoliosis targeted stretches and exercises must be performed along with patient-specific, three-dimensional corrective exercises called **"Sensorimotor Re-integration."** This method uses the automatic postural control centers in the brain which are stimulated subconsciously. Patient-specific 3-D weighting (sensorimotor re-integration) manipulates the spine and posture with necessary stimulus. Used in conjunction with customized scoliosis exercises, this routine can provide dramatic results by promoting a subconscious muscle response, both lengthening and strengthening muscles and retraining one's posture to assume a more balanced alignment to gravity. This results in stabilization, followed by a reduction of the magnitude of scoliotic curve.

All these exercises must be prescribed individually. based on size, location and rotational component of the scoliosis along with the age, flexibility, coordination and stamina of the patient. Scoliosis is different in every patient and the best scoliosis exercises must be customized to promote the best outcome.

While the scoliosis patient is strongly encouraged to participate in other forms of exercise, such as swimming, team sports, Pilates and yoga, they must not replace or inhibit scoliosis treatment or exacerbate the existing curvature. Be sure to discuss all forms of exercise and stretching with a scoliosis specialist.

Types of Muscle

For the person interested in a detailed understanding of muscles, physiology and why specific types of exercise therapy are so effective in treating scoliosis, read on!

Skeletal muscle is a form of striated muscle tissue (a form of muscle fiber clustered in parallel configurations) controlled by the somatic nervous system (associated with the voluntary control of body movements via skeletal muscles). It is one of three major muscle types; the others are cardiac (striated heart muscle) and smooth muscle (involuntary non-striated muscle). Most skeletal muscles are attached to bones by tendons. Skeletal muscle is made up of individual components known as myocytes, or "muscle cells," sometimes referred to as "muscle fibers."

Muscle fibers fall into two categories:

Type I fibers (slow to fatigue) appear red due to the presence of the oxygen-binding protein myoglobin. These fibers are suited for endurance.

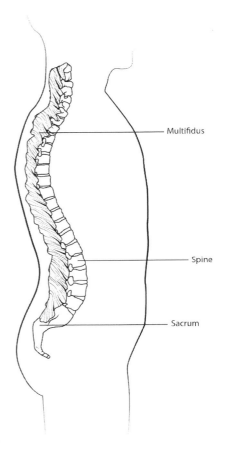

Type II fibers (fast twitch) are white due to the absence of myoglobin and a reliance on glycolytic enzymes. These fibers are efficient for short bursts of speed and power. These fibers are quicker to fatigue.

There are approximately five layers of muscle in the spine comprising superficial, intermediate and deep groups. The deepest layers control the position of each spinal vertebra. These muscles are a significantly different fiber type than the more superficial muscles in the first three layers. The deeper muscle layers are smaller, only one to three inches in length and are mainly **Type I fibers** that are fatigue resistant. Studies have demonstrated asymmetry of these muscles (**multifidus muscles**) in those with scoliosis, and they are thought to contribute greatly to the twisting and tilted individual vertebral positions in scoliosis.[125]

Muscle fiber type dictates how a muscle responds to force/load principles. These deeper spinal muscles are not under voluntary control and hence

125 "PubMed Result — NCBI." 2014. 22 Apr. 2016 <http://www.ncbi.nlm.nih.gov/pubmed?db=pubmed&cmd=link&linkname=pubmed_pubmed&uid=3249100>

NOT affected by standard isotonic exercise programs. This means that deep muscle groupings like the multifidi serve to support the body relative to gravity and also have the largest ability to alter the structural position of a single vertebrae.

Voluntary exercise programs for scoliosis like yoga and Pilates fail to stop progression, fail to reduce an existing spinal curvature, and fail to reduce the number of scoliosis curvatures progressing to surgical threshold because they do not engage this deeper muscle layer.

The immobilizing effect of old-tech scoliosis braces decreases the deep layer muscle firing, making the spine less stable and more prone to progression. In addition, poorly designed off-the-shelf scoliosis braces can create even more rotation which leads to spinal rigidity and potentially more structural asymmetry in bone and discs. New designs in scoliosis bracing are hyper-corrective. They allow and encourage the spine to move into the corrected posture, eliminating the negative muscle-damaging effects of the older brace designs. It is vital that all brace wear is accompanied by a scoliosis specific exercise program.

Spinal resistance training allows for subconscious involuntary muscle control to be affected, causing a change in the postural feedback mechanism that alter individual vertebral positions.

Spinal resistance training, using specialized scoliosis cantilevers, have demonstrated significant influence on multifidus muscles, causing less tilt and rotation of the vertebrae. The earlier a patient begins this spinal resistance training, the better the chances of permanently decreasing existing spinal curvature and halting progression.

So, if we look at the spine and how it functions, we can see that deeper muscles are shorter and more densely populated with automatic muscle fibers, ensuring upright postural stability is not lost. Superficial muscles are longer and cover greater distance, gaining mechanical advantage during movement. Therefore, posture, or "the spinal position" seen on x-ray studies, is mostly a result of intrinsic, deep automatic muscles which control the spine's position in gravity.

Automatic and not controlled by conscious signals, these muscles are not influenced by active conscious exercises, but react to specific stimulus (e.g. those that trigger a change in balance). Since the body has an existing "program" of how it aligns its center mass with gravity, and this program originates in the brain, then exercises which cause the brain to change patterns are very effective in influencing the deep automatic musculature that directly controls bone position. Sensorimotor Re-integration (by adding weight to alter body mass around the head, torso and pelvis) causes the body to reactively change its postural pattern and directs antigravity muscles to shorten and lengthen to establish a new postural balance.

By using specific x-ray and posture analysis, the doctor can measure the individual spinal units. This analysis can also demonstrate which portion of the body's alignment is furthest away from gravity, either the head, torso or pelvis. A specific amount of weight is added to a portion of the body, causing the body's reflexes to reorganize the body mass vs. gravity relationship. This reaction is subconscious. As the body reorients to gravity it creates a subconscious new body image. If done correctly, this new body scheme will have less postural distortion, less spinal rotation...less scoliosis. After several weeks, the subconscious body scheme has been altered, and the patient will stand and move differently. Posture, x-rays and function will be measurably improved.[126]

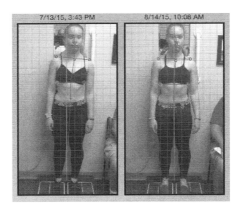

126 Gaudreault, N. "Assessment of the Paraspinal Muscles of Subjects Presenting." 2005. 23 Apr. 2016. <http://bmcmusculoskeletdisord.biomedcentral.com/articles/10.1186/1471-2474-6-14>

Chapter 31. Non-Invasive Customized Exercise for Scoliosis

Let's Look At Some Popular Non-Invasive Methods to Treat AIS (Adolescent Idiopathic Scolisosis)

Idiopathic scoliosis is the result of both genetic predisposition and specific environmental factors, which are probably interconnected. There is no one approach, adjustment or therapy which will work in every case. Therefore, treatment must be customized to the particular, specific needs of each individual patient. However, there are key aspects of any protocols which are essential to achieve consistent, measurable progress. Find a practitioner who has made scoliosis their life's work – a scoliosis specialist. Start with a more conservative approach and then work up to more invasive protocols. In consultation with an expert, start with an exercise-based program, then advance to bracing if necessary. Only as a last resort accept surgery.

The first step in developing a customized program of care involves gathering information about the biomechanical function of the entire spine – not just the area(s) affected by scoliosis. It is an *axiom* that you can control the middle of a cord by moving the top and the bottom. By the same logic, it is important to understand what is occurring in the neck and hips – the primary drivers of curve progression – in order to affect the middle of the spine. The understanding and identification of the specific environmental factors that drive idiopathic scoliosis are still poorly understood. This is called the science of epigenetics.

Potential Risk Factors for Activating Scoliosis in Those Genetically Predisposed

- Exposure to certain types of bacteria (e.g. mycobacterium)

- Minor leg length discrepancies

- Specific genetic variants

- Increased osteopontin levels

- Spinal trauma

- Poor postural habits

- Activities that cause repeated compression on the spine

- A shortened spinal cord relative to spine length

- Postural instability during a growth spurt

- Hormonal imbalances as puberty is beginning

- Neurotransmitter imbalance from nutritional deficiencies or nutritional excesses (e.g. selenium)

And many, many more….

Standard Chiropractic Treatment (non-scoliosis specialist)

Chiropractic treatment for scoliosis typically consists of spinal manipulation, isotonic exercises and shoe lifts. However, research has shown that these procedures, when applied over a one-year duration, were not sufficient to significantly reduce the Cobb angle of a scoliotic curvature. Such

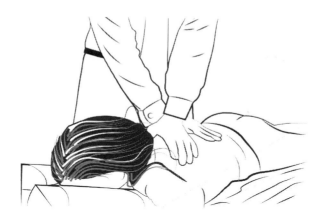

treatments alone have been shown to be largely ineffective at significantly reducing scoliotic curvatures, but can be effective in relieving pain.[127]

The CLEAR Method – An Eclectic Approach

The acronym "CLEAR" in the CLEAR Institute name stands for Chiropractic, Leadership, Educational, Advancement and Research. Established in 2000, the CLEAR Institute offers an alternative approach to the standard scoliosis treatment provided by the majority of orthopedic scoliosis specialists.[128] [129]

Though malfunctioning brains and spinal cords are suspected as part of the root cause of idiopathic scoliosis[130], the medical community still focuses on the actual curve rather than on its root cause.

---

127 Lantz, Charles A, and Jasper Chen. "Effect of Chiropractic Intervention on Small Scoliotic Curves in Younger subjects: a Time-Series Cohort Design." *Journal of Manipulative and Physiological Therapeutics* 24.6 (2001): 385-393. Print.

128 Woggon AJ, Martinez DA: Chiropractic treatment of idiopathic scoliosis: a description of the protocol. Scoliosis 2013;8(Suppl 2):P6.

129 "About CLEAR | CLEAR Scoliosis Institute." 2016. 23 Apr. 2016 <https://www.clear-institute.org/about/>

130 Burwell RG, Dangerfield PH, Grivas TB. "Scoliogeny of adolescent idiopathic scoliosis..." 2013. 4 Nov. 2016. <https://www.ncbi.nlm.nih.gov/pmc/articles/PMC3656779/>

The researchers and clinicians at the CLEAR Institute noticed a crucial discrepancy between scoliosis theory and scoliosis treatment. They developed a treatment program that focused on "retraining" the brain to "learn" how to hold the spine straighter automatically, referred to as "three-dimensional auto-correction."

A 2004 study focused on the reduction of scoliosis by manipulative and rehabilitative methods. It involved stimulation of the involuntary postural reflexes utilized in a clinic setting and at home. The results showed reduced scoliotic curvatures in 19 subjects by an average of 17 degrees within a four- to six-week period with an average reduction in Cobb angle of 62 percent. None of the patients' Cobb angles increased.[131]

As reported in Mark W. Morningstar's study, many of the proposed causes of idiopathic scoliosis are neurological.[132] They include brain asymmetry, neural axis deformities, asynchronous neurological growth and central nervous system processing errors. Also, many coexistent neurological imbalances are present in scoliosis patients, such as visual deficiency and decreased postural stability (Feise, 2001) (Lantz, 2001). Therefore, the goals of treatment are not only to reduce the scoliotic curvatures, but to rehabilitate any underlying postural and neurological weaknesses or imbalance.[133] [134] [135] [136] [137]

131 Morningstar, MW. "Scoliosis Treatment Using a Combination of Manipulative and ..." 2004. 26 Apr. 2016. <http://bmcmusculoskeletdisord.biomedcentral.com/articles/10.1186/1471-2474-5-32>

132 Burwell, R Geoffrey et al. "Whither the Etiopathogenesis (and Scoliogeny) of Adolescent Idiopathic Scoliosis? Incorporating Presentations on Scoliogeny at the 2012 IRSSD and SRS Meetings." Scoliosis 8.1 (2013): 4. 4 Nov. 2016.

133 Niesluchowski, W. "The Potential Role of Brain Asymmetry in the Development of ..." 1999. 25 Apr. 2016. <http://www.ncbi.nlm.nih.gov/pubmed/10543585>

134 Dobbs, MB. "Prevalence of Neural Axis Abnormalities in Patients with ..." 2002. 26 Apr. 2016. <http://www.ncbi.nlm.nih.gov/pubmed/12473713>

135 "PubMed Result — NCBI." 2015. 27 Apr. 2016 <http://www.ncbi.nlm.nih.gov/pubmed?db=pubmed&cmd=link&linkname=pubmed_pubmed&uid=19349194>

136 Catanzariti, JF. "Visual Deficiency and Scoliosis. — NCBI." 2001. 25 Apr. 2016. <http://www.ncbi.nlm.nih.gov/pubmed/11148645>

137 Woggon, AJ and Martinez, DA. "Changes in clinical and radiographic parameters after a regimen of chiropractic manipulation..." 2013. 4 Nov. 2016. <http://scoliosisjournal.biomedcentral.com/articles/10.1186/1748-7161-8-S1-P5>

While additional research is needed to evaluate the long-term effectiveness of the CLEAR protocols, a recent study involving 3,200 patient visits over a one-year period found that 95% of people felt the same or better immediately after CLEAR treatment, and there were no serious side effects as a result of care.[138]

The CLEAR Method of Scoliosis Treatment

The CLEAR Scoliosis Institute is an educational provider of certification and training for the **CLEAR Method** of scoliosis treatment. Doctors who provide this method must be certified by the organization. They evaluate a patient's scoliosis to determine what will successfully reduce and stabilize their spinal curvature. To begin they gauge how much resistance exists within the apical regions of the scoliosis. This rigidity of the spine is dependent on the length of time the curve has been present, the degree of rib deformation, and extent of vertebral rotation. The doctor using the CLEAR method customizes an isotonic and isometric exercise program combined with a sensorimotor re-integration program that will challenge the intrinsic spinal muscles enough to effectively reduce and stabilize the spine curvature. Spinal resistance training equipment, utilizing innovative scoliosis cantilevers, are used to apply the different forces. Theses forces cause the spine to adapt in time and in need with the result being a smaller and more stable curvature and, in cases of early intervention, the possibility of a complete elimination of diagnosable scoliosis (curves below 10 degrees).

The CLEAR approach uses spinal resistance training in conjunction with the principles of autonomic control of the spine's alignment. Some CLEAR doctors add bracing as an adjunct to their standard protocol, or scoliosis-specific exercise programs such as Schroth and SEAS.

---

138 Woggon, AJ and Woggon, DA. "Patient-reported side effects immediately after chiropractic scoliosis treatment: a cross-sectional survey utilizing a ..." Scoliosis 2015; 10:29.

"What Principles Should Guide Treatment Protocols for Scoliosis?"

First of all, the best protocols operate under the premise that scoliosis is a complex condition. Secondly, all exercise-based programs need to have a warm-up component. Patients need to warm up the soft tissues of the spine as a prelude to their exercises.

What's the best way to warm up the spine? Move! Either use the mobilizing equipment or walk. Then stretch the spine. The **Wobble Chair** (Fig. 1) provides a good spine warm-up. It sits on a ball-and-socket joint, which allows the patient to flex her spine in every direction, promoting a full range of motion. **Cervical Traction** (Figure 2) allows for active, gentle and, repetitive spinal traction), and **Vibrating Traction** uses a slow, relaxing vibration scientifically proven to relax the ligaments and soft tissues of the spine.[139] Motorized therapy tables with belts that reduce the scoliosis during the therapy further improve the mobility of the most restricted areas of the

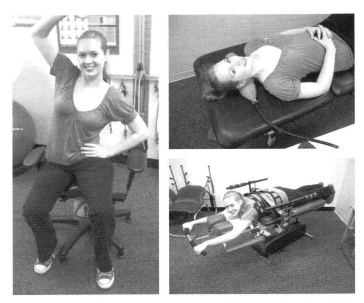

Figure 1. (left), figure 2. (right side top) and figure 3. (right side bottom)

139 Bonney, RA and Corlett, EN. "Vibration and spinal lengthening in simulated vehicle driving." 2003. 4 Nov. 2016. <https://www.ncbi.nlm.nih.gov/pubmed/12628577>

spine (Figure 3). Warming up protocols encourage the intervertebral discs to rehydrate. This reduces rigidity. Now the treatment program can more easily affect structural changes to the spine.

The **Scoliosis Traction Chair (STC)** (Figure 4) is a tool used to allow the spinal muscles to be exercised in a scoliosis-reduced position. The STC uses belting to pull the spine straight gently, traction to elongate the spine, and whole-body vibration to activate muscles.

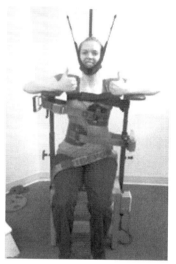 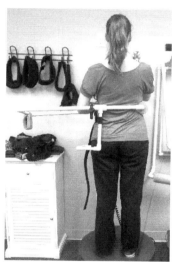

Figure 4.   *Figure 5.*

The STC is a powerful form of scoliosis therapy, and the patient must be set up in the apparatus by a knowledgeable professional who ensures that the spine is properly de-rotated.

Mechanical-adjusting instruments and a specialized therapy table enhance the precision and effectiveness of chiropractic care. These devices reduce the amount of force required to correct the spine.

In accordance with the most modern chiropractic protocols, almost all neck adjustments are performed with the use of such instruments, and the application of these adjustments are correlated with the information obtained from the patient's physical examination and x-rays.

Locking in the Changes So They Last!

Immediately after the adjustment is completed, the spine is "set" in its corrected position to ensure the permanency of the changes, also known as **Sensorimotor Re-integration (SMR)**. This involves spinal weighting protocols (typically on the head, torso and hips) and whole-body vibration therapy.[140] (Figure 5)

If the SMR protocols are not followed, any corrections achieved in the spine will be temporary. The patient will simply walk themselves back into their original distortion.

The key procedures are assembled into a home-based program of care. Isometrics, isotonics, mobilizing maneuvers, along with body weighting allow the entire program to be replicated at home with minimal equipment. The time for the home procedure varies from case to case, but typically will take one to two hours per day. It's a big commitment, but if it corrects the spine and helps a patient avoid surgery, then it's time well spent!

Follow-up Exams

Regular follow-up of the patient is critical for success. Once the custom-designed home program is either fully developed or well on its way, the scoliosis exercise specialist must again examine the patient and take a post x-ray to validate the effectiveness of the treatment protocols. This progress examination should evaluate all the findings evident on the patient's initial evaluation. Specific x-rays, which are necessary to assess correction, are limited as much as possible.

It's important to keep in mind that not all patients will show a reduction in the severity of the scoliotic curve, as measured by Cobb angle, within this time frame. This is because Cobb angle is a measurement of only two dimensions of the spine, and scoliosis is a three-dimensional condition.

---

140 Lam, TP et al., "Effect of whole body vibration (WBV) therapy on bone density and bone quality in osteopenic girls with adolescent idiopathic scoliosis …" 2013. 4 Nov. 2016. <https://www.ncbi.nlm.nih.gov/pubmed/23011683>

Before the sideways curve can be reduced or corrected, the spine must be de-rotated and decompressed in the other two dimensions. Treating a complex spinal disorder such as scoliosis is a little like reversing the path of a runaway train. It takes time to first slow down the momentum. Then more time is needed to change the course of the condition.

Home Spinal Rehab Program

The doctor and the patient need to have a frank discussion that emphasizes the importance of the patient's active participation in the treatment program. Results are not guaranteed – they are earned by patients who are willing to work alongside the doctor. The traditional methods of scoliosis treatment, bracing and surgery, are considered "passive" therapies. The patient has the procedures done to them: the doctor designs the brace, and the doctor performs the surgery. Home exercise-based programs of care, by comparison, should be considered an "active" process – the doctor teaches the patient how to do the procedures, and the patient does them. A small part of the protocols could be considered passive, but the effectiveness of these treatments on their own is limited without the involvement of the patient. The degree of patient participation affects the amount of improvement.

There's a Role For Post-surgery Exercise Programs of Care

Patients who have undergone scoliosis surgery in the past may wish to pursue an exercise-based scoliosis treatment specifically directed at the areas of the spine that have not been fused. However, these patients should not expect any degree of correction, but rather purely symptomatic relief and functional improvement (e.g., treatment to relieve their pain, improve posture and improve their activities of daily living).

It is well established that muscular atrophy undoubtedly will occur in surgically treated patients. If the muscles responsible for moving the spine are inactive for long periods of time, they will atrophy (shrink), and because rehabilitation of the muscles is a vital part of any home exercise-based scoliosis program, the patient may be unable to maintain any corrections that are achieved.

All indications are that future scoliosis treatment will focus on the underlying neuro-muscular component of the scoliotic spine and not just the symptom as measured by Cobb angle. Proactive custom-designed scoliosis exercise programs in the earliest stages of idiopathic scoliosis will be proven to be essential.

The European Schools of Scoliosis Exercise

In Europe there has developed a host of exercise-based scoliosis treatment programs. Exercise-based programs include not only the CLEAR method, but also Methode Lyonnaise, DoboMed, Functional Independent Treatment for Scoliosis (FITS), Side Shift exercises, Vojta method, Schroth (and its various offshoots), and SEAS. The **Schroth Method** is the best known of the European physiotherapeutic treatment systems, which use isometric and other exercises to strengthen and lengthen asymmetrical muscles in a scoliosis patient.

The goal of the European schools is to halt curve progression, reduce pain, increase organ capacity, partly reverse abnormal curvatures, improve posture and appearance, maintain improved posture and avoid surgery. Because these methods rely on exercises, they are limited in the permanence of the changes to the spine they can provide. Often times the treatment will be combined with bracing to get a better result.

The Schroth Method was originally designed not for adolescent idiopathic scoliosis, but instead was developed during the polio epidemics in Europe. Many of the children with polio developed a neuro-muscular form of scoliosis, and the Schroth program was designed to work on strengthening the muscles of these children. In more recent times, the program has been amended to work with AIS cases. The Schroth Method has been implemented in Europe since the 1920s. The method was developed in Germany by

Katharina Schroth, a physical therapist who had scoliosis. The method is now used in clinics specifically devoted to Schroth therapy for scoliosis patients in Germany, Spain, England and most recently in the United States.

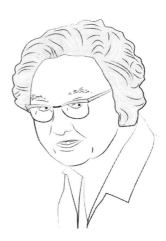

The Schroth method was further developed by Katharina Schroth's daughter, Christa Lehnert-Schroth. By the 1960s, the Schroth Method became the standard non-surgical treatment for scoliosis in Germany.

The premise behind all the European schools is that all scoliosis cases involve asymmetrical muscles. They purport that a scoliotic spine twists abnormally due to strength imbalances among muscle groups in the back and lower extremities that are supposed to be balanced. The belief is that some muscles on one side of the back grow stronger than the opposite side and pull harder on that side of the spine. The weaker muscles cannot compete, causing the asymmetry to worsen over time. Their system does not focus on underlying causes, but rather on where the "imbalance" is and how to treat it.

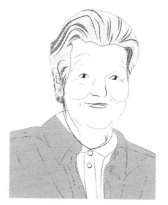

Since each individual scoliosis is unique, and exercises that benefit one patient may hinder another, an individualized exercise regime is developed to restore "balance," based on the patient's specific muscle groups that are too "weak" and "overdeveloped."

These regimens consist of muscle strengthening and stretching exercises and aim to "derotate and elongate the spine back into its normal position." The patient is required to perform these scoliosis exercises for about half an hour every day. Patient compliance is an important factor for the outcome, so they are expected to keep up with the exercises.

The principles that are applied during treatments are essentially the same for those used for the treatment of mild and moderate scoliosis cases in children, adolescents, young adults, mature adults and those with severe scoliosis. The goal of the Schroth Method scoliosis exercises is to "practice moving the body out of its unbalanced state, past the longitudinal axis toward the opposite side, until the brain is correctly reprogrammed and the patient is able to sit and stand straight upright."

Breathing techniques are used in conjunction with the exercises. The breathing instructions are believed to help push the ribs outward. The patient pushes the misaligned rib cage outward from the inside by targeted breathing against the direction in which the curved spine tends to move.[141][142]

141 "The Schroth Method — Exercises for Scoliosis." 2007. 27 Apr. 2016 <http://www.schrothmethod.com/>

142 "Scoliosis and Spinal Disorders | 10th International ..." 2016. 27 Apr. 2016 <http://scoliosisjournal.biomedcentral.com/articles/supplements/volume-8-supplement-2>

Chapter 32. Other Alternative Methods of Treatment

"Is Acupuncture A Treatment for Scoliosis?"

Traditional Chinese Medicine (TCM) therapies have been used for thousands of years to treat health problems. TCM is a system of healthcare that includes acupuncture, massage and exercises, as well as herbal medicine and syndrome-specific diets. TCM teaches that health is dependent upon an internal balance of energy forces called "yin" and 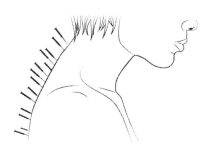 "yang." Yin represents slow passive energy in the body, and yang represents excited active energy. An imbalance of these energies promotes disease by blocking pathways, or "meridians," that allow the flow of vital energy, or "qi," throughout the body.

Acupuncture works to unblock this vital energy flow by stimulating these specific points in relation to the body's meridians. Acupuncture is used worldwide to treat pain and many other conditions. The most technologically advanced method uses a low-level laser (usually in the infrared spectrum) to stimulate the points, thereby unlocking the energy flow, relieving pain and restoring function to that specific part of the body.[143]

---

143 "Acupuncture | NCCIH." 2015. 23 Apr. 2016 <https://nccih.nih.gov/health/acupuncture>

Cold Laser Acupuncture applied at traditional acupuncture points uses low-energy laser beams instead of traditional acupuncture needles to influence the flow of current at the treatment sites. It has been shown to cause an almost identical physiologi-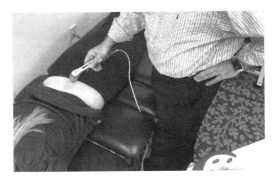cal response and brain stimulation pattern as needle acupuncture, except without any sensation. Laser acupuncture is used to treat painful conditions, headaches, arthritis, stenosis, muscle pain, as well as sinusitis and menstrual problems – even bedwetting! Practitioners of laser acupuncture have studied traditional Chinese medicine and apply these principles to point selection. They aim a beam of light from a laser tube at an acupuncture pressure point, stimulating the body the way an acupuncture needle would. The laser remains on the acupuncture point for 10 seconds to a maximum of two minutes.

Since Cold Laser has gained FDA approval with an impressive 76 percent improvement rate, Cold Lasers are now being used widely in professional sports such as the USTS Tour de France and the National Football League.

Acupuncture and Idiopathic Scoliosis

Many studies have been conducted on the use of acupuncture; however, traditional Chinese medicine diagnosis involves syndromes defined by imbalances between the body's systems, such as yin/yang deficiencies or qi stagnation, so results can be difficult to interpret in terms of western medicine. Because of these differences, very few studies exist on scoliosis and acupuncture.

One small 2008 study observed the effects of acupuncture on 24 girls between the ages of 14 and 16 with adolescent idiopathic scoliosis. Patients were divided into groups that received sessions of either "fake" acupuncture (needles placed at incorrect points) or real acupuncture treatment. Although no improvement was observed in patients with curves over 35 degrees, significant improvements were noted with the real acupuncture treatment in patients with curves that ranged from 16 to 35 degrees.[144] However, additional research is necessary to demonstrate the efficacy of acupuncture for scoliosis.

As part of my research on acupuncture as a treatment for chronic back pain, I was able to confirm that acupuncture is effective at relieving pain; it unfortunately did not improve the patient's range of movement or ability to perform their normal daily activities.[145]

At this time, insufficient evidence exists to conclusively prove the efficacy of acupuncture in the treatment of the pain associated with degenerative scoliosis, but it's likely it would be helpful. I think this is fair to say because research has shown acupuncture to be effective in areas related to pain management.[146]

Keep an open mind! No science can explain how acupuncture works, except for pain control. Many modern medical processes have not been subjected to scientific scrutiny. Surprising, but true.

144 Weiss, HR. "Acupuncture in the Treatment of Scoliosis – a Single Blind ..." 2008. 26 Apr. 2016. <http://scoliosisjournal.biomedcentral.com/articles/10.1186/1748-7161-3-4>

145 Strauss, Andrew Jay, and Charlie Changli Xue. "Acupuncture for Chronic Non-Specific Low Back Pain: A Case Series Study." *Chinese Journal of Integrated Traditional and Western Medicine* 7.3 (2001): 190-194. Print.

146 Tan, Gabriel et al. "Efficacy of Selected Complementary and Alternative Medicine Interventions for Chronic Pain." *Journal of Rehabilitation Research and Development* 44.2 (2007): 195. Print.

"Can Inversion Tables be Used for Scoliosis Treatment?"

Inversion therapy has been marketed as an alternative treatment for scoliosis. Inversion therapy involves being upside down or at an inverted angle to take gravitational pressure off the nerve roots and disks of the spine and increase the space between vertebrae for therapeutic benefits. The process is called "**inverting**." This can be done by handstands or headstands, hanging from a bar with arms at one's sides, or with an inversion machine.

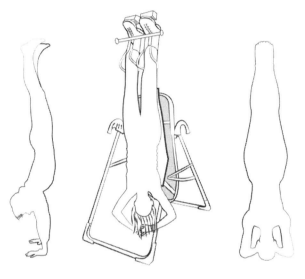

Claims

When the body's weight is suspended from the lower body the pull of gravity may decompress the joints of the body. Hanging by the feet, as with gravity boots or inversion tables, causes each joint in the body to be loaded in an equal and opposite manner to standing in an identical position of joint alignment. Inversion therapy is one example of the many ways in which spinal traction (spinal stretching) is implemented to relieve back pain.

Scoliosis Pain Relief from Inversion

Pain is not usually associated with adolescent scoliosis; therefore, most children with scoliosis are not looking for pain relief. If a child with scoliosis describes spinal pain, take them to a scoliosis specialist for an evaluation. Find out what is causing the pain.

Scoliosis Posture Correction from Inversion

Inversion therapy is promoted by some as a tool for posture correction. The increased blood flow to muscles may help to reduce back spasms. However, this will not reduce the degree of a scoliotic spine. Most current research suggests a neurological underdevelopment to be the cause of idiopathic scoliosis, that requires sensorimotor re-integration treatment.

Abdominal Strengthening

The *rectus abdominis,* or abdominal muscles, are partly responsible for the forward movement of the spine. Inversion tables can be used to perform sit-ups and crunches that strengthen these muscles. This will strengthen your core, but again it will not impact the size of your scoliosis. Scoliosis is not caused by (or as simple) as poor posture.

Research into inversion therapy and spinal traction to treat scoliosis is non-existent. Inversion therapy might bring temporary relief to scoliosis patients, but should only be considered as part of a complete treatment plan designed by your scoliosis specialist.

Possible Dangers for Scoliosis Patients

While most cases of scoliosis in children are of unknown cause, scoliosis also can result from infection, cancer, or other bony or neuromuscular diseases. Children who suffer from scoliosis as a result of these other condi-

tions should not be treated with inversion therapy unless specifically directed to do so by their scoliosis specialist.

Individuals with surgically implanted rods or supports could damage or
loosen these implanted devices during inversion.

Remember, inversion therapy is not safe for everyone!

Khan Kinetic Treatment: A New Scoliosis Therapy?

The Khan Kinetic Treatment Device (KKT-M 1) is known as a "manip-
ulator device." It's "equivalent to a similar pressure-applying device called
The Atlas Orthogonal Percussion Instrument."[147] According to the U.S.
Patent Office, the Atlas Orthogonal Percussion Instrument is used to adjust
a vertebral subluxation (dysfunctional spinal segment) of the atlas vertebra,
the top vertebra in the upper cervical spine).[148] This method of chiropractic
adjustment is based on the 1960s teachings of chiropractic developer Dr. B.
J. Palmer.[149]

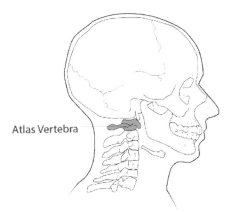

Atlas Vertebra

147 "Khan Kinetic Treatment." 2015. 27 Apr. 2016 <http://www.moh.gov.my/at-
tachments/7489.pdf>

148 "510(k) Summary — U.S. Food and Drug Administration." 2016. 27 Apr. 2016
<https://www.accessdata.fda.gov/cdrh_docs/pdf6/K060043.pdf>

149 "Chiropractic: The Palmer Method (1963) — Chirobase." 27 Apr. 2016 <http://
www.chirobase.org/05RB/BCC/11a.html>

"What is It Used For?"

The device was invented by Dr. A.H. Khan. Dr. Khan claims to treat spinal cord injury, whiplash, herniated discs, back pain, neck pain, osteoarthritis and headache. There is no independent research to back up his claims.

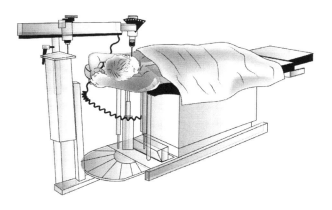

Editor's Note:

Dr. Strauss respects and uses upper cervical specific chiropractic as an integral component of a comprehensive scoliosis treatment program that centers around home-based exercise and sensorimotor re-integration. While upper cervical chiropractic (as promoted by Dr. Khan) is a powerful tool to remove nerve pressure from the spine and spinal cord, it is NOT a complete scoliosis correction program.

Dr. Strauss is a past president of the Upper Cervical Society and has studied and researched this form of specific chiropractic in great detail over the past 35 years.

Pilates for Scoliosis

Pilates is a body-conditioning routine that helps build flexibility and long lean muscles and strength and endurance in the legs, abdominals, arms, hips and back. It puts emphasis on spinal and pelvic alignment, breathing to relieve stress and allow adequate oxygen flow to muscles, developing a strong core, and improving coordination and balance.

There are books and centers dedicated to "Pilates for Scoliosis" or "Scoliosis Pilates;" however, there is no research proving the effectiveness of these programs. Though Pilates can be added to a scoliosis treatment program, it is important to discuss it first with the specialist who is treating your scoliosis, as some moves may exacerbate your curve.

Because of the complexity of scoliosis, programs like Pilates – which generally target the body's core – are not designed to correct scoliosis, but aim at stabilizing participants' back curves and reducing discomfort. It could be excellent when accompanying a custom-designed scoliosis corrective program, but inadequate if used in isolation.

Yoga for Scoliosis

Yoga's purpose is to create a balance in the body through the development of strength and flexibility. This is achieved with the ongoing practice of poses, or postures, each of which has specific physical benefits. The poses can be done quickly in succession, creating heat in the body through movement – as in vinyasa-style yoga – or more slowly to increase stamina and perfect the alignment of the pose.[150]

The poses are a constant, but the approach to them varies depending on the tradition in which the teacher was trained. Like Pilates, there are books and programs for "Yoga for Scoliosis" or "Scoliosis Yoga," but also like Pilates, the same precautions should be observed. There is no research to support its efficacy other than as a pain-management approach. Yoga will not correct scoliosis or alter its progressive nature. While there is a DVD called "Yoga for Scoliosis," its design is not to correct the scoliosis, but rather to strengthen the supportive muscles, improve flexibility and to relieve any associated pain.

---

150 "Introduction to Vinyasa Flow Yoga — Health." 2016. 27 Apr. 2016 <https://www.verywell.com/introduction-to-vinyasa-flow-yoga-3566892>

Many people hope yoga will help treat or cure idiopathic scoliosis or even believe that they can treat their scoliosis themselves. The assumption here is that scoliosis is caused by weakness. This belief is based on a misunderstanding of scoliosis in general and why the spine is curving. The current scientific literature shows that electromyography (EMG) testing goes against the assumption that scoliosis is caused by weak muscles.[151]

The muscles in scoliosis patients aren't weak; they are misdirected and uncoordinated in terms of postural control. Postural control centers are located in the brain stem and are controlled subconsciously. What this means is while one can stand up straighter through voluntary effort, an individual does NOT have direct control over how their spine orients to gravity. So, for example, when you consciously contort into a yoga pose, it does not influence the automatic posture centers of the brain. Therefore, these poses will have little to no effect on the automatic spinal muscles that pull the bones into a scoliotic curve.

These same EMG studies have shown that the very tight muscles on the outside of a scoliotic curve are actually attempting to pull the spine straighter. Therefore, there is every reason to encourage that type of muscle tightness. If you release it with yoga, you may actually increase the scoliosis.

Curve flexibility in scoliosis is primarily related to curve size and patient age. There are ways to biomechanically improve curve flexibility. By using passive stretching-mechanized therapies that primarily target the ligaments and discs on the inside part of the spinal curve, flexibility is enhanced in a targeted way. Stay away from releasing rigidity on the outside of the curve with general yoga.

That being said, yoga can be a useful component of a complete scoliosis treatment program. It also can be a fun way to encourage children and the entire family to exercise. Yoga (as any other supplemental stretching or exercise regime) MUST be used in conjunction with a full scoliosis treatment program, and there are specific precautions to adhere to. **So, PLEASE READ**

---

151 "EMG (Electromyogram) — KidsHealth." 2016. 23 Apr. 2016 <http://kidshealth.org/parent/general/sick/emg.html>

the following precautions, risks and yoga moves to stay away from if you have scoliosis.

With home exercises for any condition, it is always important to consult with your scoliosis specialist treating your condition before beginning any regimen.

> *There is much literature about scoliosis yoga and online resources with how-to guides, but this does not mean that scoliosis can be treated with yoga alone. It's important to discuss any supplementary exercise with your scoliosis doctor first to make sure it is suitable for you. Everyone's scoliosis is different; therefore, your yoga routine may need to be modified to fit your specific needs. It is never wise to attempt to treat your scoliosis on your own, even if it is a mild curve. Consult a scoliosis expert who shares your philosophy of conservative care.*

"Can Yoga Make Scoliosis Worse?"

Many patients have inquired about the benefits and risks of adding yoga to a scoliosis treatment program. The short answer is that the benefits outweigh the risks... as long as caution is taken.

Here is an overview of yoga for scoliosis and how it fits into a scoliosis stabilization and correction strategy.

There have been studies conducted that suggest activities such as ballet, competitive swimming and rhythmic gymnastics have significantly higher instances of severe scoliosis. Though it isn't clear what these activities have in common, it is believed that excessive and repeated hyperextension of the thoracic spine (mid back) or "backbending" may be the culprit. backbends have a flattening effect on the thoracic spine, which leaves the mid back more vulnerable. An article about ballet performers shows an increased incidence of scoliosis in that group.[152]

---

152 Warren, Michelle P., Gunn, JB, Hamilton, LH, Warren LF, and Hamilton, WG. (May 1986). Scoliosis and Fractures in Young Ballet Dancers. *New England Journal of Medicine*. 314, 1348-1353. doi: 10.1056/NEJM 198605223142104. 1 May 2016 http://www.nejm.org/doi/pdf/10.1056/nejm198605223142104

Some yoga-for-scoliosis postures incorporate thoracic backbends and have the potential to aggravate a patient's thoracic spinal curvature. However, this doesn't mean scoliosis patients cannot practice *yoga*, nor does it suggest that they cannot benefit from this form of exercise. **You just need to proceed with caution!**

> *Read on for the specific poses that should not be a part of your*
> **scoliosis yoga program.**

A complete scoliosis stabilization and/or reduction treatment program will consist of the following:

1. An effective method of unlocking the apex of the curvature (yoga for scoliosis can fit in here nicely).

2. An effective method of reducing the size of the curve (that does not put any other area of the scoliotic spine in jeopardy).

3. A sophisticated analysis of the posture biomechanics and adaptive patterning that will yield a program of sensorimotor retraining that will lock the new reduced curve posture in place.

Proceed with Caution!

> *Let me begin by saying I have practiced yoga for more than 40 years and remain a daily practitioner. Having completed a yoga teacher training course in 1982, certified by Kripalu Yoga (SDF) of Napa Valley in California, I have personally practiced a wide variety of yoga techniques. So, I am by no means here to demonize or vilify yoga as an exercise regimen. However, I do think it is important for those with scoliosis to read this article before beginning any classes or doing yoga at home.*

Though yoga is often recommended by well-intentioned fitness instructors and trainers, too often "scoliosis yoga" comes with counterproductive maneuvers that can make curves worse. While these moves are often very positive for normal bodies, some yoga exercises can be damaging to the scoliosis patient's progress.

Scoliosis is a peculiar condition. Each person will have a unique postural distortion.[153] Because of the complexity of curve type, size, modifiers, sagittal profiles and associated ligamentous instabilities, it is not possible for a person simply to do "scoliosis yoga." For example, you may be improving one aspect of the curve at the expense of another area of the curve. A more realistic approach is to have a specialized yoga for scoliosis program developed by a practitioner who is familiar with both yoga AND scoliosis.

When yoga is being done properly, no damage will take place, and the practitioner will be able to accomplish a specific rehabilitative goal with each posture. Yoga may have a positive effect on symptoms of scoliosis, but it will most likely not have any significant impact on halting curve progression or reducing the scoliosis spine curvature.

The type of scoliosis yoga poses that are best for you are determined by a complex equation reflecting the nature of your condition. Some movements may be contraindicated in your situation and be perfectly fine for someone else who also has scoliosis. No two scoliosis yoga patients are the same, and no one scoliosis yoga patient is ever the same twice. **YOU ARE CONSTANTLY CHANGING, AND YOUR SCOLIOSIS YOGA PROGRAM MUST CHANGE WITH YOU!**

It is also important to know that yoga for scoliosis alone can not prevent scoliosis nor can it stop its progress. You need to combine the scoliosis yoga program with professional specialized care to fully manage your condition and and treatment options. A scoliosis specialist who understands yoga (or exercise therapies generally) can determine the classification, modifiers and level of curvature in your spine and then work with you to develop an appropriate pose selection.

BEFORE starting any exercise program – whether it is yoga, Pilates, isometric, or any other exercise format, check with the physician treating you,

---

153 "Classification (King — Lenke) — Harms-spinesurgery.com." 2007. 27 Apr. 2016 <http://harms-spinesurgery.com/src/plugin.php?m=harms.SKO03P>

one who has a greater understanding of the principles stated above. If an unqualified doctor or yoga instructor suggests scoliosis yoga, please be cautious before proceeding.

Yoga Moves to Avoid

After taking all the necessary precautions into consideration and getting approval and recommendations from the practitioner treating your scoliosis, you can establish a scoliosis yoga practice. But first, here are some poses to avoid or take greater care when performing.

MINIMIZE BENDING BACKWARD WITH THE UPPER TORSO

Bending a scoliotic spine backward is cautioned against since some research has postulated it may reduce the normal front-to-back thoracic shape (kyphosis). This "normal" part of the spinal shape works to limit scoliosis progression. You want to encourage this shape, NOT do anything to reduce it! By the way... backbend positions will not effectively lessen the rib arch. There really is nothing that can. Well, surgery (possibly with rib shaving) is the only way.

The concern that back-bending postures will flatten the thoracic spine and destabilize the area can be overstated. Take it easy and reduce the backbends; in most cases you will be fine. If you notice any pain or aggravation of your scoliosis, talk it over with your scoliosis-trained yoga instructor.

Here is a list of the common back-bending poses that should be used only occasionally in a scoliosis yoga program:

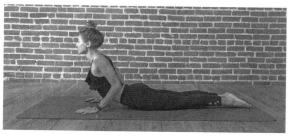

Cobra / Bhujangasana or Naga-asana

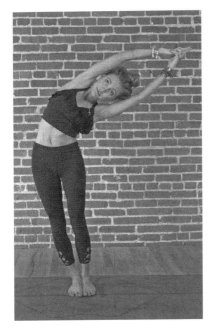
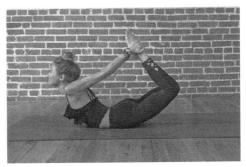
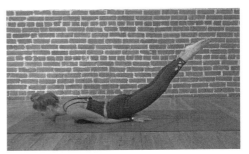

Half Moon / Ardha Chandrasana   Bow pose / Dhanurasana

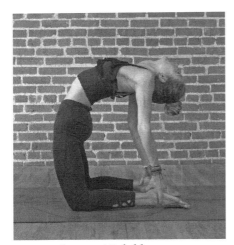
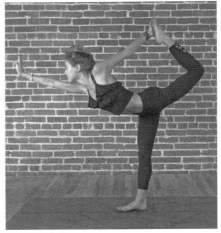

Locust / Salabhasana   *King of the Dance / Nataraja-asana*

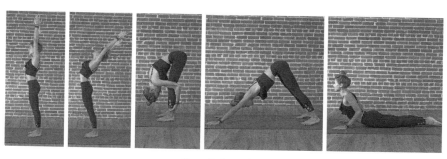

Sun Salutation

The back-bending in the Cobra or Upward Dog poses is a problem, so avoid these parts in your scoliosis yoga program. A Baby Cobra move would be a better option.

General Statement of Caution: AVOID POWER TWISTS OF THE TORSO AGAINST THE PELVIS UNLESS YOU KNOW IT WILL NOT AGGRAVATE THE RIB ARCHING.

The central segment, the rib arch, is enlarged as it rotates backward into existing curvature, regardless of whether rotation is to the left or right side. Patients with certain types of scoliosis can include these twists during their yoga for scoliosis program, BUT only to one side! Talk to your practitioner about these poses before including them in your practice. If you twist with great effort to the wrong side (or in the presence of a compensatory curve elsewhere in the spine), you are asking for trouble!

The Triangle should be avoided because the shoulder girdle is twisted against the pelvis, and the middle section must follow after the more comfortable side.

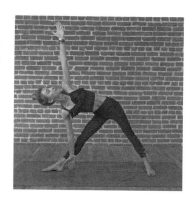

Triangle / Trikonasana

Other twisting exercises to use with caution include:

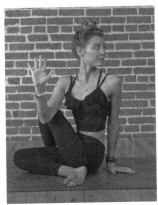 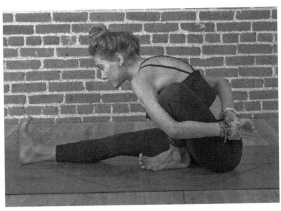

Spinal Twist / Marichyasana and the Seated Twist / Bharadvajasana

Trying to open up the main scoliotic curve between the thoracic and lumbar spine may improve the major thoracic curve, BUT at the expense of any other curvatures above or below it. How will you know that is happening? Would you be able to notice that the adjacent regions of your scoliosis were worsening?

Maybe... maybe not!

A scoliosis patient performing twisting poses to both sides would exercise into the existing curve and increase it. It is not recommended even if also performed in the opposite direction. This type of pose must be done only to one side, and if it is effective at unlocking the spine, it MUST be accompanied by sensorimotor retraining.

OTHER SCOLIOSIS YOGA EXERCISES TO AVOID:
Shoulder Stand / Sarvangasana

In the supine Shoulder Stand pose, the head is bent sharply forward at the neck. This over stretches the neck muscles. It also will promote cervical kyphosis, a reversing of the normal shape of the neck. The whole body weight is on the shoulders and may increase a rib arch formation.

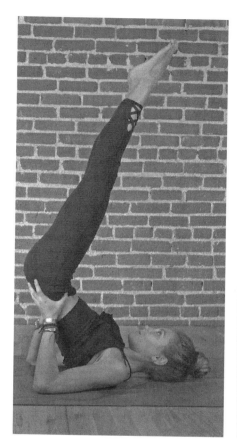
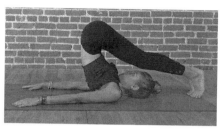
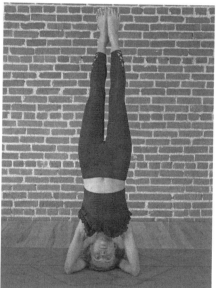

Shoulder Stand / Sarvangasana (left), The Plow / Halasana pose (top right) and The Headstand (bottom right)

An important part of any scoliosis yoga correction program is to work with improvement of the normal curvatures of the neck and low back.

Shoulder Stand will work AGAINST the establishment of normal spinal contours. Avoid it!

The Plow / Halasana pose

affects the body negatively in the same way the Shoulder Stand does. By lifting the legs up and dropping them over the torso, extreme force is applied to the spine and upper back, working against the normal neck curve.

The Headstand

A scoliotic spine is inherently weak and unstable. Turn upside down and push your spine into the skull, and you risk destabilizing it further.

The upper cervical area of the spine, the part at the top of your neck, is often problematic due to ligament stress from scoliosis.

Doing the Headstand yoga pose will place undue pressure on these weakened ligaments.

It would be better to perform isometric strengthening exercises to stabilize the weakened area.

Running

Short distance jogging and running are fine for most people with scoliosis.

Discussing fitness and exercise, the National Institute of Arthritis states:

> *"Although exercise programs have not been shown to affect the natural history of scoliosis, exercise is encouraged in patients with scoliosis to minimize any potential decrease in functional ability over time. It is very important for all people, including those with scoliosis, to exercise and remain physically fit. Girls have a higher risk than boys of developing osteoporosis (a disorder that results in weak bones that can break easily) later in life. The risk of osteoporosis is reduced in women who exercise regularly all their lives. Also, weight-bearing exercise, such as walking, running, soccer and gymnastics, increases bone density and helps prevent osteoporosis. For both boys and girls, exercising and participating in sports also improve their general sense of well-being."*[154]

Have a scoliosis specialist design or assess your running workouts. In addition to your running, a scoliosis exercise program will work to minimize

---

154 "Questions and Answers about Scoliosis in Children and ..." 2008. 27 Apr. 2016 <http://www.niams.nih.gov/Health_Info/Scoliosis/>

any negative impact of running on your scoliosis and vice versa. It also can maximize flexibility, as well as strengthen your core and hip muscles.

It is beneficial to have your gait assessed for biomechanical issues that may need to be corrected. Orthotics may be prescribed or heel lifts if a leg length discrepancy is present. Use running shoes with good cushioning to lessen impact. You can have your shoes fitted at a running store to ensure the best support.

Run on grass whenever possible for less impact on your spine. Always warm-up and stretch before your runs and cool down and stretch afterward. Stretching will help maintain spine flexibility and prevent joint stiffness. Pair your running with regular sessions with a chiropractor.

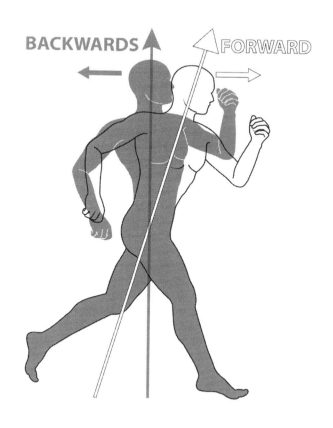

"Can 'Scoliosis Shoes' Reverse Scoliosis?"

Heel Lifts for Scoliosis

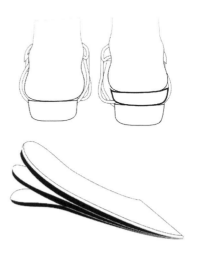

When a difference in leg lengths causes scoliosis, adding shoe wedges or lifts
to the heels may be tried. A heel lift is
a mechanical device which lengthens
the shorter leg by a prescribed amount,
thereby creating a more level platform or
base for the spine. This method works in
those rare cases where the short leg and
only the short leg is causing the scoliosis.
While a short leg is quite common among
children with scoliosis, it is also common
in the general population.

The whole picture of the scoliosis must be
looked at before reaching for a heel lift. Unfortunately, if the lift is wrongly
applied, it can make the scoliosis worse. Other considerations are pelvic rotation, abnormal shape of the sacrum, imbalance in the lower pelvis (the sit
bones), and foot pronation.

Orthotics for Scoliosis

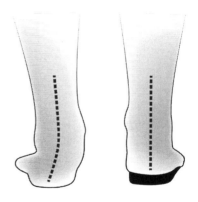

"Orthotics," "foot orthoses," "orthotic devices," or "biomechanical orthotic devices" are prescribed custom-made devices that alter the motion and change the
pressure on your feet's weight-bearing
surfaces. They allow for normal motion,
but limit abnormal motion. They can be
prescribed to help correct problems such
as excessive pronation, low arches, cavus,

high arches and painful feet. They are also prescribed after some foot operations to help maintain surgical corrections.

By altering the heel height, custom orthoses also can be used to correct a short leg, also referred to as a "leg length inequality." This can be an underlying cause of acceleration of scoliosis in some patients.

Orthopedic shoes, heel and ischial (sit bone) lifts and orthotic inserts help correct posture in some people who have skeletal abnormalities. Doctors sometimes prescribe specialized shoes and orthotic shoe inserts for people with scoliosis. These devices can help reduce associated pain and prevent further progression of the condition. Orthotics also can reduce scoliosis hip pain, scoliosis back pain, and other scoliosis back problems associated with adult scoliosis, if the pain can be attributed to a secondary orthopedic issue.

Foot Orthotics to Prevent Scoliosis

Nonstructural or functional scoliosis is a curve in the spine without rotation and is reversible because it is caused by a pain, a muscle spasm or a difference in leg length. Compensatory scoliosis is a spinal curve in the coronal plane which disappears when the patient sits. It also may be caused by either a short leg or a pelvic tilt due to contracture of the hip.

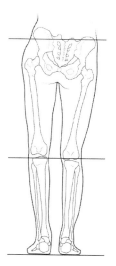
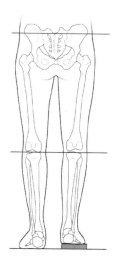

An asymmetrical leg growth could result in imbalanced spinal growth. Using a heel lift – a wedge-shaped shoe insert – in the shoe of the shorter leg can add extra support and promote more balanced spinal growth. However, if one leg is shorter because the foot has poor arch development or because the child places excess weight on the inside of one sole, they may require a custom orthotic to support the foot in the areas around the arch. If the leg is functionally, rather than anatomically, shorter, the scoliosis may worsen if a heel lift is used rather than an orthotic shoe insert.

Research on Foot Orthotics

An article published in a 2001 issue of *European Spine Journal*, showed adolescent patients with scoliosis that had significantly reduced spinal curvature and improved postural adaptations (e.g. better pelvis alignment) after wearing shoe lifts.[155]

Orthopedic shoes and custom foot orthotics may prevent further progression of certain types of scoliosis in children with asymmetrical legs and reduce back pain in adults with scoliosis. However, whether heel lifts can reduce existing spine curvature is still to be determined. More research remains to be done to clarify the use of orthotics in the treatment of scoliosis. By taking an x-ray with the orthotic in place, it can be determined how the orthotic is affecting the scoliotic spine.

---

155 Zabjek, KF. "Acute Postural Adaptations Induced by a Shoe Lift in ... — NCBI." 2001.19 April 2016 http://www.nejm.org/doi/pdf/10.1056/nejm198605223142104 <http://www.ncbi.nlm.nih.gov/pubmed/11345630>

> *"Whenever I write about mental health and integrative therapies, I am accused of being prejudiced against pharmaceuticals. So let me be clear – integrative medicine is the judicious application of both conventional and evidence-based natural therapies."*
>
> **– Andrew Weil**

Chapter 33. Can Scoliosis be Cured Naturally?

Let's Take a Look at Homeopathy and Holistic Practices and Their Purported Treatment of Scoliosis

Holistic medicine (from the Greek *holos*, meaning *all, whole, entire, total*) is a form of alternative medicine that considers the whole person (body, mind, spirit and emotions) in terms of health and wellness. Holistic medicine operates under the principle that optimal health is dependent upon proper balance in life.

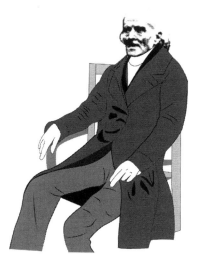

Practitioners of holistic medicine believe that people are comprised of interdependent parts, and if one part is not working properly, all the other parts will be affected. This will create imbalances (physical, emotional, or spiritual) and thus negatively affect overall health.[156]

---

156 "Holistic Medicine: What It Is, Treatments ... — WebMD." 2012. 27 Apr. 2016 <http://www.webmd.com/balance/guide/what-is-holistic-medicine>

Homeopathy (from the Greek *hómoios* "like" + *páthos* "suffering"), also known as homeopathic medicine, is one of the most popular holistic systems of medicine. It was developed more than 200 years ago by the German physician Samuel Hahnemann. According to his doctrine *similia similibus curentur* ("like cures like"), a substance that causes the symptoms of a disease in a healthy person will cure similar symptoms in sick people.[157]

> **Before we explore the use of homeopathy, let's set the record straight…. While many people swear by homeopathic remedies and use them regularly as their primary health care, mostresearch has found them to be ineffective and their purported benefits implausible. So, in spite of the huge number of advocates in the general community, the majority of the scientific community regards homeopathy as placebo care.**

An Overview of Homeopathic Treatments and the Many Adherents Who Swear by These Unusual Remedies:

The National Center for Complementary and Alternative Medicine states:

> *"Supporters of homeopathy point to two unconventional theories: 'like cures like' – the notion that a disease can be cured by a substance that produces similar symptoms in healthy people; and 'law of minimum dose' – the notion that the lower the dose of the medication, the greater its effectiveness. Many homeopathic remedies are so diluted that no molecules of the original substance remain.*
>
> *Homeopathic remedies are derived from substances that come from plants, minerals, or animals, such as red onion, arnica (mountain herb), crushed whole bees, white arsenic, lead, mercury, poison ivy, belladonna (deadly nightshade), and stinging nettle. Homeopathic remedies are often formulated as sugar pellets to be placed under the tongue; they may also be in other forms, such as ointments, gels, drops, creams, and tablets. Treatments are 'individualized' or tailored*

---

157 "Homeopathy — Wikipedia, the Free Encyclopedia." 2011. 27 Apr. 2016 <https://en.wikipedia.org/wiki/Homeopathy>

to each person – it is not uncommon for different people with the same condition to receive different treatments."

The Status of Homeopathy Research

The research on homeopathy collectively has concluded that there is little evidence to support homeopathy as an effective treatment for any specific condition, including scoliosis.

It has been difficult to perform research on homeopathy because the key concepts of it are not consistent with fundamental principles of chemistry and physics. How would it be possible to explain in scientific terms how a remedy containing little or no active ingredient can have any effect. This has led to major challenges to rigorous clinical investigation of homeopathic remedies. For example, one cannot confirm that a remedy works when it has been diluted to the point that not even one molecule of the original substance is in the bottle!

Another research challenge is that homeopathic treatments are highly individualized, and there is no uniform prescribing standard for homeopaths. There are hundreds of different homeopathic remedies, which can be prescribed in a variety of different dilutions to treat thousands of symptoms.

Homeopathic Treatment for Scoliosis

Here is a statement from a leading homeopathic organization on Scoliosis care.

"The selection of remedy is based upon the theory of individualization and symptoms similarity by using holistic approach. This is the only way through which a state of complete health can be regained by removing all the sign and symptoms from which the patient is suffering. The aim of homeopathy is not only to treat scoliosis but to address its underlying cause and individual susceptibility."[158]

In my opinion there is no scientific support for this statement.

---

158 "Scoliosis — Disease Index, Musculo-Skeletal — Hpathy.com." 2011. 27 Apr. 2016 <http://hpathy.com/cause-symptoms-treatment/scoliosis/>

Various Scoliosis Remedies from the World of Alternative or Holistic 'Medicine'

Editor's Note: While Dr. Strauss believes herbal treatments may provide muscle relaxation, he does not think they correct scoliosis.

Herbal Oils

Individual oils of thyme, oregano, cypress, birch, basil, peppermint and marjoram are used in herbal oil treatments.

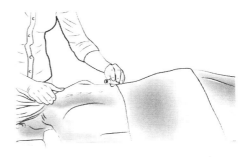

It is reputed that repeated application once a month will produce some realignment of the spine in cases of scoliosis.

Some believe aromatherapy combined with massage application will produce "a surge of energy" that is helpful. They believe oils deliver a frequency of energy, building on each other.[159]

Bach Flowers

Bach flowers are primarily used for emotional imbalances. There are 38 flower remedies that were discovered in the 1930s by the late Dr. Edward Bach.

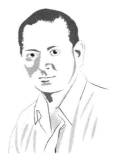

Since then they have been used by many doctors, homeopaths and other healthcare professionals around the world, who have reported successful treatments with babies, children, adults and animals.

---

159 "What Are the Treatments for Mild Scoliosis? | eHow." 2009. 27 Apr. 2016 <http://www.ehow.com/facts_5006530_what-treatments-mild-scoliosis.html>

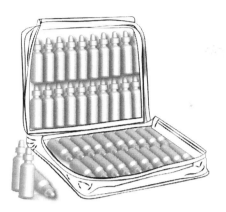

Rescue Remedy is the most well known bach flower. It is used to treat shock.[160]

---

160 "Scoliosis and Bach Flowers — Alternative ..." 2007. 27 Apr. 2016 <http://scoliosis.homestead.com/bachflowers.html>

Chapter 34. Clothing Choices

Approximately 12 percent of females suffer from scoliosis, and many of them are adolescent girls. Scoliosis can cause visible symptoms: uneven shoulders, head held off center, ribs at different heights, a shoulder blade that sticks out more than the other, uneven hips, one leg appearing shorter than the other, or the body leaning to one side.

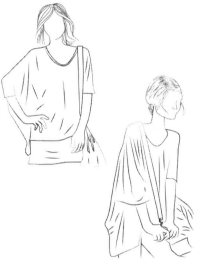

Severe cases will present with more visible symptoms.

Because scoliosis causes asymmetry in the body, ill-fitting clothing may be an everyday problem. The waist on pants or skirts may appear uneven, or shirts and dresses may not fit or hang on the body properly. Dressing in a way that makes the individual feel best and secure with their scoliosis can become a challenge.

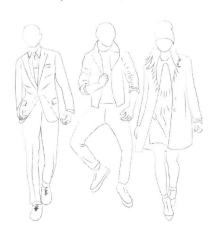

One of the easiest ways to mask scoliosis is to avoid tight-fitting clothes. Individuals with scoliosis tend to be small framed and long waisted, so their bones are very pronounced. Tight shirts make asymmetry more obvious, and lopsided tightness is uncomfortable. This can even lead to aches by the end of the day.

So, if masking these asymmetries in the hips or shoulders is your goal, then looser clothing such as shawls, cardigans, hoodies, blazers and jackets should be your go-to styles. Luckily, current fashion includes wearing over-sized billowy T-shirts over tanks and layering cardigans and sweaters.

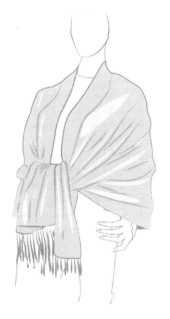

If you feel too insecure to wear a strappy sundress tank top or camisole alone, then a light denim jacket or sweater thrown over top looks nice and can allow you the freedom to wear those items without feeling too exposed. There are many lightweight material options available. Even a Pashmina can be a quick and versatile option.

If it's a high hip that concerns you, then a nice wide bag can balance the difference. These do not have to be large or heavy, which will only cause pain over time. Many bags come in lightweight materials, so take the time to find the right one.

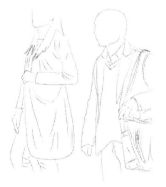

Smock and babydoll dresses are in fashion now, and compared to more fitted styles they offer coverage without being unflattering or boring.

For discrepancies in pant leg lengths, the [best option is to buy pants that fit your longest leg the best and then hem the other side. This is an inexpensive alteration that a tailor can do. If you are frugal, doing the sewing yourself is a cost-effective option.

Dresses and skirts can look uneven at the hem for someone with scoliosis. A seamstress can pin the hem up to look straight while the skirt is on. Then later, she can stitch the new hem into place at a machine or by hand. It'll look uneven on a hanger, but that's OK. When worn the new hem will give the illusion that the clothes are straight.

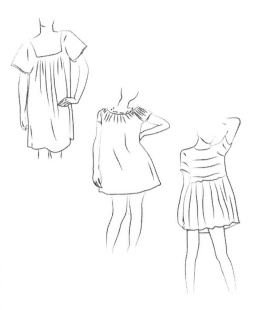

The most important thing is to be confident in who you are and how you feel. Many people have scoliosis including famous models, athletes and actresses (e.g., actress Shailene Woodley, actress and model Rebecca Romijn, Olympics track star Usain Bolt, cellist Yo-Yo Ma, and actress and singer Vanessa Williams).

You are probably more aware of your physical traits than others, so if you truly want others not to notice, then you must carry yourself as if there is no difference. People respond to confidence. If you carry yourself with self-confidence, that is what people will pay attention to – not your scoliosis!

Conclusion: Now It's Your Turn!

You've already seen the testimonials of many scoliosis sufferers who have had significant improvements in their conditions after exercise-based scoliosis treatment.

Why not let that be your story?

You're Standing At a Crossroads...
Which Way Will You Choose?

You have three options.

1. Your first option is to do nothing. This takes you down a tortuous road of pain, frustration and embarrassment as you try to deal with your scoliosis instead of fighting it and getting your life back.

2. Your second option is to take the advice of your ortho doctor. He or she will either ask you to wear outdated and ineffective braces – *prepare for dangerous spinal fusion surgery with risk of complications later in life* – or ask you to give up your hard-earned money for treatments, which only give you temporary relief at best.

3. The third option is to try a custom-designed, home-based exercise program designed specifically for scoliosis. With a home exercise-based scoliosis treatment system, you finally can fight your scoliosis and take back control of your life.

Which sounds like the **BEST OPTION** to you?

Remember, waiting longer will only give more opportunity for scoliosis curves to worsen! But, exercise-based scoliosis treatment has been **PROVEN to WORK**.

WHY NOT let it work for **YOU**?

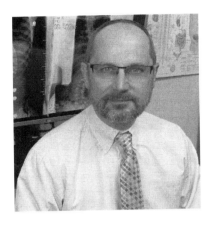

Yours in health,

Dr. Andrew Strauss, BS, DC, MS

P.S. Remember that all severe scoliosis curves have one thing in common; they started out as mild curves and progressively got worse. Do something about your child's scoliosis N-O-W and reclaim control over your family's life. I have treated scoliosis curves ranging from mild to severe and patients from age 7 to age 83, but the sooner you start intensive scoliosis treatment, the better the results will be.

So make that leap of faith today.

FAQs

We understand that you may have questions about the effectiveness of this treatment for your particular situation. Please take a look at our frequently asked questions below. If you don't find the answer to your questions, your CLEAR Institute certified doctore would be happy to answer them. "My scoliosis has already progressed significantly. Is it too late for treatment?"

"My scoliosis has already progressed significantly. Is it too late for treatment?"

No. While early intervention before the progression of curves is always preferable, we have seen patient after patient reduce their curves and experience relief from their pain and disability using these exercises. We may only be able to modestly straighten your spine, but significant postural and cosmetic changes are still very likely.

We understand the pain and helplessness you feel, but there is something you can do about your condition. Don't watch your curves progress for a single day longer than you already have.

"I have a mild curve. Do I qualify for treatment?"

Yes. Patients with a curvature(s) of less than 25 degrees with mild degeneration and low pain levels respond the best to exercise-based programs of care. All severe curves have one thing in common: they all started as mild curves. There is great potential for you to reduce pain and the risk of further progression and even reverse the curve you already have. The best time to treat scoliosis is before progression, severe degeneration or pain.

"I have a severe curve. Do I qualify for treatment?"

Yes. Patients with a curvature(s) of more than 25 degrees require longer treatment because rigidity and compensations have complicated the scoliosis. While it is always preferable to begin intervention before scoliosis progresses, it is never too late to begin your treatment. Most will see results within weeks.

"Does the CLEAR Institute methods treat all ages?"

Yes. Our youngest patient right now is 7 years old and our oldest is 83. No matter what age or stage you are experiencing, the time to prevent further progression and reduce the risk of pain and disability is now.

"Can I receive treatment if I do not live in the area?"

Yes. CLEAR Institute intensive certified doctors   Offer special one to four-week intensive treatment plans that work effectively when combined with at-home exercises. This approach is ideal for out-of-town guests. Many patients visit intensive certified doctors from all over the country and the world. Don't let location be the only obstacle to receiving the treatment that will change your life forever. Call today to arrange your customized treatment plan.

- Directions
- Accommodations (We have two Hilton hotels next door. They typically offer our patients discounted rates.)
- Travel and US Visa assistance

Don't let location be the only obstacle to receiving the treatment that will change your life forever. Call us today to arrange your customized treatment plan.

"What if it doesn't work?"

What do you have to lose by giving the home exercise-based solution a try? There are:

- No risks of making your pain or progression worse
- No scars
- No ineffective, "old technology" back braces
- No more feeling like there is nothing you can do

"I would like to speak with the doctor directly to decide if this solution is right for me. May I?"

Of course! Of course! The contact details for the CLEAR Institute are:

Email: care@clear-institute.org
Phone: (866) 663-7030
Fax: (612) 545-3230

You will directed to the doctor who is right for you.

Works Cited

"510(k) Summary — U.S. Food and Drug Administration." 2016. Web. 27 Apr. 2016. <https://www.accessdata.fda.gov/cdrh_docs/pdf6/K060043. pdf>

"About CLEAR | CLEAR Scoliosis Institute." 2016. Web. 23 Apr. 2016. <https://www.clear-institute.org/about/>

"Acupuncture | NCCIH." 2015. Web. 23 Apr. 2016. <https://nccih.nih.gov/ health/acupuncture>

Adobor, RD. "School Screening and Point Prevalence of ... — NCBI." 2011. Web. 18 Apr. 2016. <http://www.ncbi.nlm.nih.gov/pmc/articles/ PMC3213177/>

"Adults with Idiopathic Scoliosis Improve Disability ... — Springer." 2016. Web. 11 Apr. 2016. <http://link.springer.com/content/pd-f/10.1007%2Fs00586-016-4528-y.pdf>

Akazawa, Tsutomu et al. "Corrosion of Spinal Implants Retrieved from Patients with Scoliosis." *Journal of Orthopaedic Science* 10.2 (2005): 200-205. Print.

Allred, CC. "Successful Use of Noninvasive Ventilation in Pregnancy." 2014. Web. 25 Apr. 2016. <http://err.ersjournals.com/content/23/131/142. full.pdf>

Beauchamp, Marc et al. "Diurnal Variation of Cobb Angle Measurement in Adolescent Idiopathic Scoliosis." *Spine* 18.12 (1993): 1581-1583. Web. 18 Apr. 2016.

Bonney, RA and Corlett, EN. "Vibration and spinal lengthening in simulated vehicle driving." 2003. Web. 4 Nov. 2016. <https://www.ncbi.nlm. nih.gov/pubmed/12628577>

Burwell, R Geoffrey et al. "Whither the Etiopathogenesis (and Scoliogeny) of Adolescent Idiopathic Scoliosis? Incorporating Presentations on

Scoliogeny at the 2012 IRSSD and SRS Meetings." *Scoliosis* 8.1 (2013): 4. Web. 4 2016.

Burwell, RG. "Adolescent Idiopathic Scoliosis (AIS), Environment ..." 2011. Web. 25 Apr. 2016. <http://scoliosisjournal.biomedcentral.com/articles/10.1186/1748-7161-6-26>

Burwell, RG. "Scoliogeny of Adolescent Idiopathic Scoliosis: Inviting ..." 2013. Web. 4 Nov. 2016. <http://scoliosisjournal.biomedcentral.com/articles/10.1186/1748-7161-8-8>

Calvo-Muñoz, Inmaculada, Antonia Gómez-Conesa, and Julio Sánchez-Meca. "Prevalence of Low Back Pain in Children and Adolescents: a Meta-Analysis." *BMC Pediatrics* 13.1 (2013): 1. Web.18 Apr. 2016.

"Can you be Allergic to Spine Hardware? | Dr. Stefano ..." 2014. Web. 25 Apr. 2016. <http://sinicropispine.com/can-allergic-spine-hardware/>

Canavese, F. "Serial Elongation-Derotation-Flexion Casting for Children with ..." 2015. Web. 25 Apr. 2016. <http://www.ncbi.nlm.nih.gov/pmc/articles/PMC4686440/>

"Casting and Traction Treatment Methods for Scoliosis (PDF ..." 2015. Web. 21 Apr. 2016. <https://www.researchgate.net/publication/5900787_Casting_and_Traction_Treatment_Methods_for_Scoliosis>

Catanzariti, JF. "Visual Deficiency and Scoliosis. — NCBI." 2001. Web. 25 Apr. 2016. <http://www.ncbi.nlm.nih.gov/pubmed/11148645>

"CDC — Ergonomics and Musculoskeletal Disorders — NIOSH ..." 2003. Web. 20 Apr. 2016. <http://www.cdc.gov/niosh/topics/ergonomics/>

"Chiari Malformation Fact Sheet." 2006. Web. 23 Mar. 2016. <http://www.ninds.nih.gov/disorders/chiari/detail_chiari.htm>

"Chiropractic — Mission of the World Chiropractic Alliance." Web. 20 Apr. 2016. <http://www.worldchiropracticalliance.org/>

"Chiropractic: The Palmer Method (1963) — Chirobase." Web. 27 Apr. 2016. <http://www.chirobase.org/05RB/BCC/11a.html>

"Classification (King — Lenke) — Harms-Spinesurgery.com." 2007. Web. 27 Apr. 2016. <http://harms-spinesurgery.com/src/plugin.php?m=harms.SKO03P>

"CLEAR Scoliosis Institute." 2011. Web. 26 Apr. 2016. <https://www.clear-institute.org/>

"Clinical Laboratory Improvement Amendments (CLIA ..." 2005. Web. 21 Apr. 2016. <https://www.cms.gov/clia/>

"Cobb Angle — Wikipedia, the Free Encyclopedia." 2011. Web. 31 Mar. 2016. <https://en.wikipedia.org/wiki/Cobb_angle>

Cole, D., Ilharreborde, B., Woo, R. (2015) Retrospective Cost Effectiveness Analysis of Implanet Jazz Sublaminar Bands for Surgical Treatment of Adolescent Idiopathic Scoliosis. Web. 23 Apr. 2016. <http://www.im-planet.com/wp-content/themes/theme-implanet/pdf/Health_Advances_Jazz_Cost-Effectiveness.pdf>

Dastych, M. "Changes of Selenium, Copper, and Zinc Content in Hair and ..." 2008. Web. 25 Apr. 2016. <http://www.ncbi.nlm.nih.gov/pubmed/18404661>

Dastych, M. "Idiopathic Scoliosis and Concentrations of Zinc ... — NCBI." 2002. Web. 25 Apr. 2016. <http://www.ncbi.nlm.nih.gov/pubmed/12449234>

Deckey, Jeffrey E., and David S. Bradford. "Loss of Sagittal Plane Correction after Removal of Spinal Implants." *Spine* 25.19 (2000): 2453-2460. Print.

"Die Skoliose in ihrer Behandlung und Entstehung nach ..." 2013. Web. 20 Apr. 2016. <http://www.worldcat.org/title/skoliose-in-ihrer-behandlung-und-entstehung-nach-klinischen-und-experimentellen-studien/oclc/21218666>

Dietz, V. "Proprioception and Locomotor Disorders — UFJF." 2002. Web. 25 Apr. 2016. <http://www.ufjf.br/especializacaofisioto/files/2013/06/Proprioception-and-locomotor-disorders.pdf>

Dobbs, MB. "Prevalence of Neural Axis Abnormalities in Patients with ..." 2002. Web. 26 Apr. 2016. <http://www.ncbi.nlm.nih.gov/pubmed/12473713>

Drza-Grabiec, J. "Effects of the Sitting Position on the Body Posture of ... — NCBI." 2015. Web. 26 Apr. 2016. <http://www.ncbi.nlm.nih.gov/pubmed/24962297>

"EMG (Electromyogram) — KidsHealth." 2016. Web. 23 Apr. 2016. <http://kidshealth.org/parent/general/sick/emg.html>

"Evaluation of Back Pain in Children and Adolescents ..." 2009. Web. 11 Apr. 2016. <http://www.aafp.org/afp/2007/1201/p1669.html>

Fayssoux, RS. "A history of Bracing for Idiopathic Scoliosis in North America." 2010. Web. 20 Apr. 2016. <http://www.ncbi.nlm.nih.gov/pubmed/19462214>

Frigerio, E. "Metal Sensitivity in Patients with Orthopaedic Implants: a ..." 2011. Web. 26 Apr. 2016. <http://www.ncbi.nlm.nih.gov/pubmed/21480913>

Gaudreault, N. "Assessment of the Paraspinal Muscles of Subjects Presenting." 2005. Web. 23 Apr. 2016. <http://bmcmusculoskeletdisord.biomedcentral.com/articles/10.1186/1471-2474-6-14>

"Gene CHD7 linked with Scoliosis [Archive] — National ..." 2009. Web.15 Apr. 2016. <http://www.scoliosis.org/forum/archive/index.php/t-8938.html>

"Genetic Scoliosis Research — Texas Scottish Rite Hospital ..." 2013. Web.15 Apr. 2016. <http://www.tsrhc.org/genetic-scoliosis-research>

Goldberg, CJ. "Adolescent Idiopathic Scoliosis: the Effect of Brace Treatment ..." 2001. Web. 26 Apr. 2016. <http://www.ncbi.nlm.nih.gov/pubmed/11148644>

Götze, C. et al. "[Long-term Results of Quality of Life in Patients with Idiopathic Scoliosis after Harrington Instrumentation and their Relevance for Expert Evidence]." *Zeitschrift fur Orthopadie und ihre Grenzgebiete* 140.5 (2001): 492-498. Web.18 Apr. 2016.

Grivas, TB. "SOSORT Consensus Paper: School Screening for ... — NCBI." 2007. Web. 26 Apr. 2016. <http://www.ncbi.nlm.nih.gov/pmc/articles/PMC2228277/>

Guo, J. "A Prospective Randomized Controlled Study on the Treatment ..." 2014. Web. 26 Apr. 2016. <http://link.springer.com/article/10.1007%2Fs00586-013-3146-1>

Hahn, Frederik, Reinhard Zbinden, and Kan Min. "Late Implant Infections Caused by Propionibacterium Acnes in Scoliosis Surgery." *European Spine Journal* 14.8 (2005): 783-788. Print.

Hawes, M.C. (2002). *Scoliosis and the Human Spine.* Tucson, Arizona: West Press. Print.

Hershkovich, O. "Association Between Body Mass Index, Body Height ... — NCBI." 2014. Web. 26 Apr. 2016. <http://www.ncbi.nlm.nih.gov/pubmed/24332597>

"Holistic Medicine: What It Is, Treatments ... — WebMD." 2012. Web. 27 Apr. 2016. <http://www.webmd.com/balance/guide/what-is-holistic-medicine>

"Homeopathy — Wikipedia, the Free Encyclopedia." 2011. Web. 27 Apr. 2016. <https://en.wikipedia.org/wiki/Homeopathy>

Huh, S. "Cardiopulmonary Function and Scoliosis Severity in ... — NCBI." 2015. Web. 26 Apr. 2016. <http://www.ncbi.nlm.nih.gov/pmc/articles/PMC4510355/>

"Index of Paper_pdf — Osteopathic Research Web." 2012. Web. 20 Apr. 2016. <http://www.osteopathic-research.com/paper_pdf/>

"Infantile Scoliosis — Medscape Reference." Web. 23 Mar. 2016. <http://emedicine.medscape.com/article/1259899-overview>

"Introduction to Vinyasa Flow Yoga — Health." 2016. Web. 27 Apr. 2016. <https://www.verywell.com/introduction-to-vinyasa-flow-yoga-3566892>

Jackson, R. "The Classic: The Cervical Syndrome — NCBI — National ..." 2010. Web. 26 Apr. 2016. <http://www.ncbi.nlm.nih.gov/pmc/articles/PMC2881998/>

Ji, X et al. "Change of Selenium in Environment and Risk of Adolescent Idiopathic Scoliosis: a Retrospective Cohort Study." *Eur Rev Med Pharmacol Sci* 17.18 (2013): 2499-503. Web. 21 Apr. 2016.

Jokar, M. "Epidemiology of Vasculitides in Khorasan Province, Iran." 2015. Web. 26 Apr. 2016. <http://www.ncbi.nlm.nih.gov/pmc/articles/PMC4487463/>

Jones, G. "PMC PDF — NCBI — National Institutes of Health." 2005. Web. 26 Apr. 2016. <http://www.ncbi.nlm.nih.gov/pmc/articles/PMC1720304/pdf/v090p00312.pdf>

Jones, GT., and GJ Macfarlane. "Epidemiology of Low Back Pain in Children and Adolescents." *Archives of Disease in Childhood* 90.3 (2005): 312-316. Web.18 Apr. 2016.

"Jules Guérin – Wikipedia." Web. 26 Apr. 2016. <https://sv.wikipedia.org/wiki/Jules_Gu%C3%A9rin>

Jull, GA. "Motor Control Problems in Patients with Spinal Pain: a New ..." 2000. Web. 26 Apr. 2016. <http://www.ncbi.nlm.nih.gov/pubmed/10714539>

"Khan Kinetic Treatment." 2015. Web. 27 Apr. 2016. <http://www.moh.gov.my/attachments/7489.pdf>

Kim, HD. "Electron Microprobe Analysis and Tissue Reaction ... — NCBI." 2007. Web. 26 Apr. 2016. <http://www.ncbi.nlm.nih.gov/pmc/articles/PMC2857498/>

Knott, Patrick et al. "SOSORT 2012 Consensus paper: Reducing X-ray Exposure in Pediatric Patients with Scoliosis." *Scoliosis* 9.1 (2014): 1. Web. 21 Apr. 2016.

Kruse, LM. "Polygenic Threshold Model with Sex Dimorphism in ... — NCBI." 2012. Web. 26 Apr. 2016. <http://www.ncbi.nlm.nih.gov/pubmed/22992817>

Kulis, Aleksandra et al. "Participation of Sex Hormones in Multifactorial Pathogenesis of Adolescent Idiopathic Scoliosis." *International Orthopaedics* 39.6 (2015): 1227-1236. Web. 19 Apr. 2016.

Labelle, H. "Screening for Adolescent Idiopathic Scoliosis: an ... - NCBI." 2013. Web. 26 Apr. 2016. <http://www.ncbi.nlm.nih.gov/pmc/articles/PMC3835138/>

Lam, TP et al., "Effect of whole body vibration (WBV) therapy on bone density and bone quality in osteopenic girls with adolescent idiopathic scoliosis ..." 2013. Web. 4 Nov. 2016. <https://www.ncbi.nlm.nih.gov/pubmed/23011683>

Lantz, Charles A, and Jasper Chen. "Effect of Chiropractic Intervention on Small Scoliotic Curves in Younger Subjects: a Time-Series Cohort Design." *Journal of Manipulative and Physiological Therapeutics* 24.6 (2001): 385-393. Print.

"Lenke Classification System for Scoliosis | Lawrence Lenke ..." 2012. Web. 24 Mar. 2016. <http://spinal-deformity-surgeon.com/a-leader-in-spinal-deformity/lenke-classification-system-for-scoliosis/>

"Lumbar Fusion | University of Maryland Medical Center." Web. 26 Apr. 2016. <http://umm.edu/programs/spine/health/guides/lumbar-fusion>

Mahmood, SS. "The Framingham Heart Study and the Epidemiology ... — NCBI." 2014. Web. 25 Apr. 2016. <http://www.ncbi.nlm.nih.gov/pmc/articles/PMC4159698/>

Modi, HN. "Scoliosis and Spinal Disorders | Pre-publication history ..." 2009. Web. 26 Apr. 2016. <http://www.scoliosisjournal.com/content/4/1/11/prepub>

Morningstar, MW. "Scoliosis Treatment Using a Combination of Manipulative and ..." 2004. Web. 26 Apr. 2016. <http://bmcmusculoskeletdisord.biomedcentral.com/articles/10.1186/1471-2474-5-32>

Negrini, A. "Scoliosis-Specific Exercises can Reduce the Progression of ..." 2015. Web. 26 Apr. 2016. <http://www.ncbi.nlm.nih.gov/pmc/articles/PMC4537533/>

Negrini, S. "Why do we Treat Adolescent Idiopathic Scoliosis ... — NCBI." 2006.Web. 22 Apr. 2016. <http://www.ncbi.nlm.nih.gov/pubmed/16759352>

Niesluchowski, W. "The Potential Role of Brain Asymmetry in the Development of ..." 1999. Web. 25 Apr. 2016. <http://www.ncbi.nlm.nih.gov/pubmed/10543585>

Oh, CH. "A Comparison of the Somatometric Measurements of ... — NCBI." 2014. Web. 26 Apr. 2016. <http://www.ncbi.nlm.nih.gov/pubmed/23511644>

Orvomaa, E. "Pregnancy and Delivery in Patients Operated by the ... — NCBI." 1997. Web. 26 Apr. 2016. <http://www.ncbi.nlm.nih.gov/pubmed/9391799>

Pace, Nicola, Leonardo Ricci, and Stefano Negrini. "A Comparison Approach to Explain Risks Related to X-ray Imaging for Scoliosis, 2012 SOSORT award winner." *Scoliosis* 8.11 (2013): 7161-8. Web.19 Apr. 2016.

Page, P. "Cervicogenic Headaches: an Evidence-Led Approach ... — NCBI." 2011.Web. 26 Apr. 2016. <http://www.ncbi.nlm.nih.gov/pubmed/22034615>

"Patient Controlled Analgesia (PCA) Pumps: The Basics." 2015. Web. 25 Apr. 2016. <http://www.ppahs.org/2012/05/patient-controlled-analgesia-pca-pumps-the-basics/>

"Patients and Families — Scoliosis Research Society." 2015. Web. 25 Mar. 2016. <https://www.srs.org/persian/patient_and_family/scoliosis/index.htm>

"Paul Randall Harrington — Wikipedia, the Free Encyclopedia." 2011. Web. 26 Apr. 2016. <https://en.wikipedia.org/wiki/Paul_Randall_Harrington>

"PubMed Result — NCBI." 2014. Web. 22 Apr. 2016. <http://www.ncbi.nlm.nih.gov/pubmed?db=pubmed&cmd=link&linkname=pubmed_pubmed&uid=3249100>

"PubMed Result — NCBI." 2014. Web. 26 Apr. 2016. <http://www.ncbi.nlm.nih.gov/pubmed?link_type=MED_NBRS&access_num=3182881&cmd=Link&dbFrom=PubMed&from_uid=3182881>

"PubMed Result — NCBI." 2015. Web. 27 Apr. 2016. <http://www.ncbi.nlm.nih.gov/pubmed?db=pubmed&cmd=link&linkname=pubmed_pubmed&uid=19349194>

"Questions and Answers about Scoliosis in Children and ..." 2008. Web. 27 Apr. 2016. <http://www.niams.nih.gov/Health_Info/Scoliosis/>

Ramírez, M. "Body Composition in Adolescent Idiopathic Scoliosis — NCBI." 2013. Web. 26 Apr. 2016. <http://www.ncbi.nlm.nih.gov/pmc/articles/PMC3555626/>

Ramírez, Manuel et al. "Body Composition in Adolescent Idiopathic Scoliosis." *European Spine Journal* 22.2 (2013): 324-329. Print.

Ramírez, Norman et al. "Back Pain During Orthotic Treatment of Idiopathic Scoliosis." *Journal of Pediatric Orthopaedics* 19.2 (1999): 198-201. Print.

Ramirez, Norman, Charles E. Johnston, and Richard H. Browne. "The Prevalence of Back Pain in Children Who Have Idiopathic Scoliosis*." *J Bone Joint Surg Am* 79.3 (1997): 364-8. Web.18 Apr. 2016.

Reamy, Brian V., and Joseph B. Slakey. "Adolescent Idiopathic Scoliosis: Review and Current Concepts." *American Family Physician* 64.1 (2001). Print.

Reamy, BV. "Adolescent Idiopathic Scoliosis: Review and Current Concepts." 2001. Web. 26 Apr. 2016. <http://www.ncbi.nlm.nih.gov/pubmed/11456428>

Renshaw, T. S. "The Role of Harrington Instrumentation and Posterior Spine Fusion in the Management of Adolescent Idiopathic Scoliosis." *The Orthopedic Clinics of North America* 19.2 (1988): 257-267. Print.

Reynolds, RA. "Postoperative Pain Management after Spinal Fusion Surgery ..." 2013. Web. 26 Apr. 2016. <http://www.ncbi.nlm.nih.gov/pubmed/24436846>

"Rib Vertebral Angle in Scoliosis | Bone and Spine." 2013. Web. 25 Mar. 2016. <http://boneandspine.com/rib-vertebral-angle-in-scoliosis/>

"Risks and Long-Term Complications of Adolescent Idiopathic ..." 2013. Web. 26 Apr. 2016. <http://www.oapublishinglondon.com/article/498>

Rullander, AC. "Young People's Experiences with Scoliosis Surgery: a Survey ..." 2013. Web. 26 Apr. 2016. <http://www.ncbi.nlm.nih.gov/pubmed/24247313>

Rullander, Anna-Clara et al. "Young People's Experiences with Scoliosis Surgery: a Survey of Pain, Nausea, and Global Satisfaction." *Orthopaedic Nursing* 32.6 (2013): 327-333. Print.

Sahay, M. "Rickets – Vitamin D Deficiency and Dependency — NCBI." 2012. Web. 26 Apr. 2016. <http://www.ncbi.nlm.nih.gov/pmc/articles/PMC3313732/>

Saunders, Travis J, Jean-Philippe Chaput, and Mark S Tremblay. "Sedentary Behaviour as an Emerging Risk Factor for Cardiometabolic Diseases in Children and Youth." *Canadian Journal of Diabetes* 38.1 (2014): 53-61. Print.

Schimmel, JJP. "Adolescent Idiopathic Scoliosis and Spinal Fusion do not Substantially ..." 2015. Web. 26 Apr. 2016. <http://www.ncbi.nlm.nih.gov/pmc/articles/PMC4459442/>

"Scoliosis – Disease Index, Musculo-Skeletal – Hpathy.com." 2011. Web. 27 Apr. 2016. <http://hpathy.com/cause-symptoms-treatment/scoliosis/>

"Scoliosis | Wunderkammer." 2012. Web. 20 Apr. 2016. <http://wunderkammer.ki.se/images/scoliosis>

"Scoliosis and Bach flowers – Alternative ..." 2007. Web. 27 Apr. 2016. <http://scoliosis.homestead.com/bachflowers.html>

"Scoliosis and Spinal Disorders | 10th International ..." 2016. Web. 27 Apr. 2016. <http://scoliosisjournal.biomedcentral.com/articles/supplements/volume-8-supplement-2>

"Scoliosis Causes & Types (Structural & Nonstructural)." 2007. Web. 24 Mar. 2016. <http://www.webmd.com/back-pain/tc/scoliosis-cause>

"Scoliosis Research Society." 2015. Web. 25 Apr. 2016. <https://www.srs.org/chinese_sim/patient_and_family/the_aging_spine/pseudarthrosis.htm>

"Scoliosis Surgery: Things to Consider-OrthoInfo — AAOS." 2011. Web. 25 Apr. 2016. <http://orthoinfo.aaos.org/topic.cfm?topic=A00641>

"ScoliScore Genetic Test for Progressive Scoliosis ..." 2012. Web. 26 Apr. 2016. <http://scoliosisnj.com/scoliscore/>

Sengupta, DK. "Scoliosis – The Current Concepts." 2010. Web. 26 Apr. 2016. <http://www.ncbi.nlm.nih.gov/pmc/articles/PMC2822419/>

Shang, X. "Metal Hypersensitivity in Patient with Posterior Lumbar Spine ..." 2014. Web. 25 Apr. 2016. <http://bmcmusculoskeletdisord.biomedcentral.com/articles/10.1186/1471-2474-15-314>

Shang, Xianping et al. "Metal Hypersensitivity in Patient with Posterior Lumbar Spine Fusion: a Case Report and its Literature Review." *BMC Musculoskeletal Disorders* 15.1 (2014): 314. Print.

Siegel, JA. "The Birth of the Illegitimate Linear No-Threshold Model: An ..." 2015. Web. 26 Apr. 2016. <http://www.ncbi.nlm.nih.gov/pubmed/26535990>

"Spinal Fusion: MedlinePlus Medical Encyclopedia." 2006. Web. 26 Apr. 2016. <https://www.nlm.nih.gov/medlineplus/ency/article/002968.htm>

"SpineCor Dynamic Corrective Brace." 2013. Web. 22 Apr. 2016. <http://www.spinecor.com/ForProfessionals/SpineCorDynamicCorrective-Brace.aspx>

Strauss, Andrew J., and Charlie Changli Xue. "Acupuncture for Chronic Non-Specific Low Back Pain: A Case Series Study." *Chinese Journal of Integrated Traditional and Western Medicine* 7.3 (2001): 190-194. Print.

Syazwan, A. "Poor Sitting Posture and a Heavy Schoolbag as ... – NCBI." 2011. Web. 26 Apr. 2016. <http://www.ncbi.nlm.nih.gov/pubmed/22003301>

Tan, Gabriel et al. "Efficacy of Selected Complementary and Alternative Medicine Interventions for Chronic Pain." *Journal of Rehabilitation Research and Development* 44.2 (2007): 195. Print.

"The History of Lumbar Spine Stabilization." 2005. Web. 26 Apr. 2016. <http://www.burtonreport.com/infspine/SurgStabilSpineHistory.htm>

"The Schroth Method – Exercises for Scoliosis." 2007. Web. 27 Apr. 2016. <http://www.schrothmethod.com/>

Thyssen, Jacob Pontoppidan et al. "The Association Between Metal Allergy, Total Hip Arthroplasty, and Revision: A Case-Control Study." *Acta Orthopaedica* 80.6 (2009): 646-652. Print.

Timgren, J. "Reversible Pelvic Asymmetry: an Overlooked ... – NCBI." 2006. Web. 26 Apr. 2016. <http://www.ncbi.nlm.nih.gov/pubmed/16949945>

"Transgenomic – ScoliScore AIS Test." 2015. Web. 21 Apr. 2016. <http://www.transgenomic.com/services/genetic-testing/scoliscore-ais-test/>

"Transgenomic – ScoliScore." 2015. Web.15 Apr. 2016. <http://www.transgenomic.com/product/scoliscore/>

Tsiligiannis, T. "Pulmonary Function in Children with Idiopathic Scoliosis | Scoliosis and ..." 2012. Web. 26 Apr. 2016. <http://scoliosisjournal.biomedcentral.com/articles/10.1186/1748-7161-7-7>

Tsiligiannis, Theofanis, and Theodoros Grivas. "Pulmonary Function in Children with Idiopathic Scoliosis." *Scoliosis* 7.1 (2012): 7. Web. 22 Apr. 2016.

Vasiliadis, ES. "Historical Overview of Spinal Deformities in Ancient Greece ..." 2009. Web. 26 Apr. 2016. <http://scoliosisjournal.biomed-central.com/articles/10.1186/1748-7161-4-6>

Warren, Michelle P., Gunn, JB, Hamilton, LH, Warren, LF, and Hamilton, WG. (May 1986). Scoliosis and fractures in young ballet dancers. *New England Journal of Medicine.* 314, 1348-1353. doi: 10.1056/NEJM 198605223142104. Web. 1 May 2016. <http://www.nejm.org/doi/pdf/10.1056/nejm198605223142104>

Weiner, MF. "Abstract – Nature Publishing Group." 2009. Web. 26 Apr. 2016. <http://www.nature.com/sc/journal/v47/n6/abs/sc200919a.html>

Weinstein, SL. "Effects of Bracing in Adolescents with Idiopathic ... – NCBI." 2013. Web. 20 Apr. 2016. <http://www.ncbi.nlm.nih.gov/pmc/articles/PMC3913566/>

Weinstein, SL. "Health and Function of Patients with Untreated ... – NCBI." 2003. Web. 26 Apr. 2016. <http://www.ncbi.nlm.nih.gov/pubmed/12578488>

Weinstein, SL. "PubMed – NCBI." 2008. Web. 26 Apr. 2016. <http://www.ncbi.nlm.nih.gov/pubmed/18456103>

Weiss, Hans-Rudolf, and Deborah Goodall. "Rate of Complications in Scoliosis Surgery – a Systematic Review of the PubMed Literature." *Scoliosis* 3.1 (2008): 1. Web. 22 Apr. 2016.

Weiss, HR, and Goodall, D. "Rate of Complications in Scoliosis Surgery – a Systematic... – NCBI." 2008. Web. 26 Apr. 2016. <http://www.ncbi.nlm.nih.gov/pmc/articles/PMC2525632/>

Weiss, HR. "Acupuncture in the Treatment of Scoliosis – a Single Blind ..." 2008. Web. 26 Apr. 2016. <http://scoliosisjournal.biomedcentral.com/articles/10.1186/1748-7161-3-4>

Weiss, HR. "Adolescent Idiopathic Scoliosis – to Operate or Not? A ... – NCBI." 2008. Web. 26 Apr. 2016. <http://www.ncbi.nlm.nih.gov/pmc/articles/PMC2572584/>

"What Are the Treatments for Mild Scoliosis? | eHow." 2009. Web. 27 Apr. 2016.<http://www.ehow.com/facts_5006530_what-treatments-mild-scoliosis.html>

Wick, JM. "Infantile and Juvenile Scoliosis: The Crooked Path to ..." 2009. Web. 25 Apr. 2016. <http://www.aornjournal.org/article/S0001-2092(09)00551-1/abstract>

Woggon, AJ and Martinez, DA. "Changes in clinical and radiographic parameters after a regimen of chiropractic manipulation..." 2013. Web. 4 Nov. 2016. <http://scoliosisjournal.biomedcentral.com/articles/10.1186/1748-7161-8-S1-P5>

Woggon, AJ and Martinez, DA. "Chiropractic treatment of idiopathic scoliosis: a description of the protocol." Scoliosis (2013); 8(Suppl 2): 6. Print.

Woggon, AJ and Woggon, DA. "Patient-reported side effects immediately after chiropractic scoliosis treatment: a cross-sectional survey utilizing a ..." Scoliosis (2015); 10:29. Print.

Worthington, V. "Nutrition as an Environmental Factor in the Etiology of ... – NCBI."1993. Web. 26 Apr. 2016. <http://www.ncbi.nlm.nih.gov/pubmed/8492060>

Zabjek, KF. "Acute Postural Adaptations Induced by a Shoe Lift in... – NCBI." 2001. Web. 19 Apr. 2016. <http://www.ncbi.nlm.nih.gov/pubmed/11345630>

Zaina, F. "Adolescent Idiopathic Scoliosis and Eating Disorders: is ..." 2013. <http://www.ncbi.nlm.nih.gov/pubmed/23357674> Web. 25 Apr. 2016.